BRAIN EXERCISES

BRAIN EXERCISES TO CURE ADHD

Amnon Gimpel, M.D.
Psychiatrist and Neurologist

Contributions by:
Lynn Gimpel, Ph.D.
Brain physiology and pharmacology

Avigail Gimpel, M.S.
Learning disabilities and ADHD

Typeset in Arno Pro by Koren Publishing Services

Library of Congress Control Number: 2007908888

BookSurge Publishing
North Charleston, South Carolina

Contents

Acknowledgements

Many people made contributions to this book and I want to thank each of them at this time.

First and above all, I would like to thank my wife who has supported all my projects and endeavors. This book has been a labor of love for both of us and she has been an active participant and best advisor and critic of each chapter. In addition to contributing the material on brain physiology and pharmacology, she has read and corrected most pages in this book. In depth research in all areas helped me present to the reader the most recent information about ADHD some of which is still in press.

The couples that are featured in this book, we saw together as co-therapists of the Marriage and Sex Counseling Clinic at Emory University School of Medicine or in private practice.

My son, Micah, spent many nights helping organize the material in a format that moved the project forward. His advice and constant questioning was needed and appreciated.

My daughter in law, Avigail, in addition to her valuable contribution about learning disabilities, was very helpful in providing constructive criticism which improved the content as well as the selection of case histories and examples.

A special thanks goes to Dr. Shaya Wexler who helped shape the direction of the book and gave me many valuable suggestions all of which I incorporated into this book.

Many friends and colleagues spent hours reading the first version of the text and literally transformed the book with their insight and suggestions. The book is much clearer and more practical as a result of their input. Dr. Lois Feinerman and Dr. Chaim Heitner spent many hours reviewing the text in detail. Talia Roth was one of the first who took on the project of reading the rough draft and opened my eyes to how much work needed to be done.

It has been a pleasure to work Liron Tal at TCD Design and Chaya Mendelson at Koren Publishing Services.

I want to thank my son who allowed me to tell his story from grade school to the present as he coped and overcame ADHD. He is amazing.

My patients, colleagues and teachers have influenced this book in countless ways. I am indebted to them.

Introduction

ADHD, or Attention Deficit Hyperactivity Disorder, is a problem that has become increasingly prevalent in the past decade. The terms ADHD and ADD are used to describe the same condition and therefore I will use ADHD exclusively. In the early years of trying to describe the syndrome, some scientists emphasized the attention deficit and some emphasized the hyperactivity; different individuals have varying degrees of symptoms but all suffer from inattention. The American Psychiatric Association combined these terms when it was clear they are the same. The difficulty with this particular disorder is that, despite being recognized more easily by professionals in recent years, most physicians and therapists do not have a long-term solution. Medication, such as Ritalin, cannot solve the problems associated with ADHD alone, nor does it result in any permanent changes in the brain. As soon as Ritalin use is stopped, the symptoms of ADHD return. Now, however, new techniques and strategies, targeted mental and physical exercises have been proven to reduce and even permanently eliminate the symptoms of ADHD in children, teenagers and adults. Despite what some may think, ADHD is a *thinking* disorder and not a behavioral one. It is *not* because the child is lazy or spoiled and it is *not* because of poor parenting. Targeted mental and physical exercises can increase neuronal connections in the brain. These connections strengthen the brain and increase its flexibility and acuity. Even better, these methods are totally natural and designed to eliminate the need for medication over time.

Mental and physical exercises combined learning techniques for problem solving, planning ahead and reflection, work *together* to increase neuronal connections. The more neurons connected to each other to support a given function, the stronger the impulse. The more neurons recruited, the more total neurotransmitter even though the deficit at each synapse still exists. For example, as a result of vigorous brain stimulation, each neuronal synapse incorporates many more neurons to support the same function. Therefore, the total *concentration* of neurotransmitter is many times higher to send a much stronger signal. This strengthens the brain dramatically.

This ground breaking comprehensive approach comes from my personal and professional experiences and has been refined and enriched by brilliant research from world class institutions over the past few years. We are all indebted to them. Any treatment short of this is really behind the times. I am shocked at how often I find treatment used in the early 80s and 90s that continue to be recommended by professionals as if nothing transpired since they graduated. Medical knowledge often doubles every 10 years; you should expect medical treatment to follow right behind new advances. The research that has been done in the last few years will have a profound effect on how we treat memory loss, learning disabilities, psychological difficulties, ADHD, brain injury and a host of other disabilities. If the Nobel Prize is based on the number of people whose quality of life will be greatly improved, then this revolutionary breakthrough in brain neurophysiology will be worthy of one.

ADHD is now a major concern for parents, school officials

and professionals. Despite the fact that medication relieves many of the symptoms, fear and uncertainty continue to plague many parents. A lack of accurate information and unsatisfactory results cause many parents to avoid medical treatment and professional help. Even with positive results, parents are uncomfortable with medicating a young child every day.

This book will relieve the uncertainty. Up to date information is the key to fully understanding the cause of ADHD and common sense practical strategies can be implemented for effective treatment.

Childhood, adolescent and adult ADHD are all similar disorders but need to be approached differently. In the following chapters, we will address the best ways to achieve optimal neurological function in each of these categories and stages of life. By sharing true stories about patients and my own and my family's personal history, I will show how to implement specific treatment as years go by.

After having spent most of my professional life seeing thousands of cases and studying the latest techniques with new insight into the cause and cure of ADHD, I am confident that when you implement this new approach to treatment, very positive results will follow.

In the early 1990s, parents and medical professionals around the world noticed an alarming increase in the number of children diagnosed with the symptoms of Attention Deficit Disorder (ADD). Difficulties at home and the persistent complaints from school officials caused many parents to look for help. Discovered in 1956, methylphenidate (Ritalin) proved to be a very effective treatment. Although it produced dramatic results over a wide patient base in thousands of children, parents were highly resistant to it and resented continuously medicating their children. Some were suspicious that it was a plot by drug manufacturers and the medical community to make money. Some imagined it was a condition invented by the medical profession and pharmaceutical companies. There were claims of side effects such as addictive properties or inhibiting the growth of the child. Others thought it was a result of environmental pollution. Perhaps, some said, medication would interfere with creativity or other talents. No one could fathom why there seemed to be a sudden increase in the number of children who were being diagnosed as hyperactive or unable to stay focused.

These same accusations and complaints were duplicated in Israel beginning in 2000. Many Israelis felt that the condition was highly exaggerated and over-diagnosed or was a result of over-crowded schools, poor teachers or parenting. The fact is that ADHD is under-diagnosed, not over-diagnosed, especially in adults. It is also often misdiagnosed by tests that give a large number of false positives. We have concrete proof of the cause, we know exactly where the deficit is in the brain, and we are learning how to treat it very effectively.

The only way to dispute all the unfounded claims, accusations and suspicions is for the parents to familiarize themselves with the most recent research and findings in the etiology and treatment of ADHD. Then they can decide the truth for themselves. There is definitely a place for Ritalin in many cases. But it does not solve the problem and does *not* result in any permanent changes in the brain. Ritalin is useful to temporarily relieve the symptoms of ADHD, but parents and teachers should known that this is a short term solution to help the student until treatment aimed at permanent changes in brain function produces results. Mental and physical brain exercises make permanent changes by raising the concentration of neurotransmitters at the synapse for a calmer, more focused person. The information we have today about the adaptability and plasticity of the human brain has revolutionized the prognosis for many mental and also physical disabilities. For those suffering from ADHD, this has led to the development of mental and physical exercises as well as problem solving techniques and other additional strategies that have been shown to "build a better brain" and can diminish or eliminate ADHD symptoms as well as the use of Ritalin

ADHD is quite prevalent. It is a relatively minor glitch in the function of the most complex organ on earth. When parents learn that their child has ADHD, they commonly experience multiple conflicting emotions – relief to have an answer behind their child's behavior and to learn that it is not imagined, fear of what awaits them in the future, and confusion as to how to handle it.

When parents ask for help dealing with their out of control children, they want immediate strategies to ensure that their child would excel both emotionally and academically. But before parents can help their child overcome his challenges and fulfill his potential, they must understand what ADHD really means. What exactly is ADHD?

Until very recently, we didn't have the answer to this question. The prefrontal lobes of the brain, behind the forehead, have been identified as the region of the brain responsible for decision-making, emotional responses, critical thinking and all the more sophisticated mental functions.

Studies have shown that this area of the brain does not function adequately in ADHD patients because there are not enough active neurotransmitters at the synapses in the frontal lobes. These chemicals in the brain are responsible for the transmission of information necessary to manage attention, concentration and impulsivity. This includes emotional monitoring, energy levels, agitation, motor movements and tremor. As a result of this deficiency in neurotransmission, children with ADHD will have difficulties in some or all of these areas. To a casual observer, the child appears immature for his age. Adults and society in general have expectations of age appropriate behavior. For example, if a child of 7 behaves in school or socially as if he were 5, you can predict what the results will be. If a child of 17 has the brain maturity of 13, there will be consequences in all areas from social and academic to relationships with family members and failure to meet expectations.

If the part of the brain responsible for emotional decisions is not working effectively, emotional reactions will often be inappropriate or irrational, too extreme or understated. It is more difficult both to get over anger and to separate emotions from one situation to the next. Often these emotions are carried around for the rest of the day and released at events or on people totally unrelated to the initial episode.

Understanding that there is a biological deficit at the root of ADHD is a necessary precondition in order for us to understand why medication reduces the symptoms and why specific targeted brain exercises are so effective in stimulating permanent brain growth and development.

There are completely natural ways to correct this in the vast majority of cases. The development of these lagging skills is not rocket science. It takes commitment, practice, persistence and more practice. Any skill requires dedicated practice, including sophisticated thinking skills. If you want to play the piano or learn a new language or play a great game of tennis, you will have to invest time and effort. ADHD requires the same commitment.

Teachers and parents who embrace the new treatment methods will see very positive changes in focus, concentration, impulse control, thinking skills and school performance. Both parents and teachers can incorporate these exercises into the activities of daily living and *learning. The goal is to empower parents and enable their child to improve brain function without the slightest chance it will have any detrimental effect at all.* The fact is that the kind of training that needs to be done intensively with ADHD children would benefit anyone.

It is encouraging and inspiring to hear about famous people who led successful lives without any treatment at all for ADHD symptoms, but the reality is that the vast majority of ADHD sufferers have great difficulty reaching their potential. Not until the '80's was a full set of symptoms for this condition described. The goal is to move your child into the category that would be described as very successful and enable your child to reach his potential.

Personal History

In my family, I can trace four generations that displayed varying degrees of ADHD, including myself in the second generation. This has given me a close personal perspective and an even better understanding of my patients over the past 35 years. My training as an American Board Certified psychiatrist and neurologist, as well as my own struggles with this condition, gave me an enduring interest in ADHD.

My mother, who spoke five languages, had a university degree in pharmacy and worked as one of the first pharmacists in Israel, had classic ADHD symptoms. One can succeed professionally even with the limitations of ADHD and no treatment or even diagnosis. Of course, during the 1940s and 50s, this condition was not defined although the symptoms of ADHD were clearly exhibited.

Living with my mother was stressful. As a hospital pharmacist she had to interact with only a few people as most medication was dispensed only to the hospital staff. This profession suited her because her social skills were never fully developed. These poor social skills impacted me continuously.

A situation that occurred frequently involved our holiday

trips together as a family. Very few people had cars in the '40s and '50s so the use of public transportation was necessary every time we traveled out of town. The thought of traveling with my mother by bus caused me a great deal of anxiety because most of our trips ended in a major embarrassment. Her undeveloped social skills, impulsivity and volatile temper always caused an argument with the driver or one of the passengers. Her lack of sensitivity also caused endless conflicts. Comments such as "Don't sit next to that person. His clothes are dirty." or "The driver must be from Africa because he's so dark" were commonplace with her. My mother would often hold running conversations so disorganized that the original topic was completely lost. The person she was talking to, usually a total stranger, would stare with a look of total confusion or shock. Before it was all over, I always felt that the passengers were looking at me with pity.

There was endless conflict with our extended family. It reached a point where we hardly saw them. People were always hurt or offended by her comments and she was often oblivious to social cues. Despite the fact that she was highly educated, she had very poor organization and planning skills.

My father did his best to keep our house in a minimum state of order. He worked very long hours and so was unable to entirely compensate for her lack of organization. Frequently in the morning, I could not find clean clothes to wear to school. When I could find them, they were usually in a completely different and unexpected part of the apartment.

Often my mother would return from the market with only half the items needed to prepare supper. My father soon took over meal planning and the shopping. When my father had to work late, my brother and I would go to the nearest fast food stand for dinner. It's fortunate that the food we liked was relatively healthy food because it was certainly a staple of our diet.

There were also regular fights with neighbors over minor issues. I don't think there was a single neighbor with whom she had a good relationship. She went through life with very few friends or social ties and made many foolish financial mistakes because of impulsive decisions. She always seemed to buy at the top and sell at the bottom.

I remember her developing habits to try to help herself. She carried a notebook with her all the time full of 'to do' lists. There was a schedule for every goal that she set for herself and she referred to it many times during the day. However, the notebook had another purpose. She studied languages continuously and wrote down new words every day. Learning languages was really a form of brain stimulation that was therapeutic. She must have received some relief from the ADHD symptoms by improving her thinking skills and reducing painful symptoms.

She also had an enormous amount of energy and was always on the move. I don't have a memory of my mother just sitting quietly. She talked all the time and was in constant motion. At a bus stop or in a store, she would strike up conversations with strangers, especially new immigrants who just arrived in Israel, as a way to improve her language skills and channel her energy.

However, when it came to her children, she always expressed strong love and confidence in us. Even though I was a very poor student, she always reminded me of my few good grades and when talking to others in my presence, always praised me. I was well aware of my poor performance, but her praise and encouragement for any accomplishment allowed me to feel good about myself. It seems to me she understood that I had many problems in school but did not seem able to take the steps to prepare for the future. However she did focus on my accomplishments and build my confidence. I knew that I was not the best student in the class. She didn't talk about who was the best student; only about how smart she thought I was. She constantly told me what a wonderful boy I was and how proud she was of me. My brother and I always knew that our mother loved us and we were sure no other kid in the neighborhood was loved as much as we were. This was one of the strongest feelings I carried through childhood.

Since my home was so disorganized, I never had a specific place to study. However, it is quite likely that even with a desk I would have been overwhelmed by homework assignments. As a child in grade school and high school, all I hoped for was to pass to the next grade. I hated school. Many mornings I used to go to my father with symptoms of illness. I had stomach pains or a headache or some other complaint. My father understood my anxiety and usually said to me, "Try to go to school and if you continue to feel bad during the day, I will come get you." It was easier with my mother. She often would let me stay home. Staying home did not make me happy or help me but when I knew I didn't have to go to school, I always felt better.

I could seldom finish my homework. I "found" many excuses; I was too busy with sports and as a scout youth movement leader. Nevertheless, I found a solution. I would arrive 30 minutes before class and my friends would help me. Many kids did the same, but for me, it was a way of life, a system of compensation.

In school, before certain classes or with certain teachers, I felt panic. If I was called upon to read in front of the class, my weaknesses would be exposed. No teacher was ever mean to me, but to read in front of the class was a terrible ordeal. I developed a strategy to help myself. To reduce the probability that the teacher would call on me, I would always ask questions during the class and participate in answering the questions even when I didn't know the answer. The teachers wanted everyone to participate during class so if I took an active role then, it reduced the probability that she would call on me to read. I simply could not stay connected and was always losing the place where I needed to read. The strategy worked! As a result, I reduced a major stress during school.

One time I asked my mother for help with homework. Her response was very positive and I was able to complete the assignments. She was very patient and loving despite the fact it took hours to finish. Her comment at the end of this grueling task was,

"You see how smart you are. We finished everything in only two hours." However, her help with homework was really beyond her ability to tolerate on a regular basis and it was soon dropped.

Emotional support did not alleviate my ADHD symptoms but my mother's loving attitude was much more important than anything else. Her constant praise gave my brother and me self esteem, confidence and a strong emotional foundation

My last year in high school was by far the most difficult and stressful year of my life. From the beginning of the year, I was stressed about the matriculation exams at the end of the year. But like most children with ADHD, I took no real steps as far as planning. I could not seem to organize a schedule to help me review all the material. I continued with all my sports activities, playing soccer for our high school team as well as playing soccer in an organized youth league. At the same time, I continued to be a senior scout youth leader as if no exams awaited me at the end of the year.

Four months before exam time, my older brother asked me about my preparation for the exams. I told him that I hadn't even started. He was shocked and reviewed my school situation with my parents. He concluded that I could not possibly pass the exams without tutors in numerous areas of study. My parents were unprepared for this and unable to afford the cost. My brother, who was working at the time, offered to finance most of the expenses.

For the rest of the year I would ride my bicycle to the homes of five different tutors after school. I stopped all my sport and youth activities and studied all day long and far into the night. I would fall asleep exhausted, but routinely would wake up in a cold sweat after a terrible nightmare. The nightmare was always the same. I failed the exams because I did not know the material or because the time ran out before I could finish.

When I took the exams at the end of the year, I barely passed. Since that day, if I am under stress, the same nightmare returns.

The examiner calls for the papers and I was not able to finish answering the questions.

As a child I was able to overcome many of the symptoms of ADHD and I treated myself by finding after school activities where I could excel. Although grade school and high school were extremely difficult for me in areas of concentration, reading, homework and organization, I was very fortunate that, by the time I completed high school with great difficulty, I had more or less outgrown many of the symptoms and was able to overcome the handicaps of many years of under-performance. In the '50s in Israel, treatment was simply not an option. I recognized my limitations and turned to other areas where I could succeed such as sports and leadership positions in youth groups. This, along with a loving family, was crucial in building my self esteem and confidence.

After army service, I went to the United States for college. I had only basic English skills. The tremendous effort it took to learn English while in college was accomplished by taking math and science courses in the first year where the English was a lesser necessity. Of course I was not aware that studying English was strengthening many other areas of my brain. I have no doubt that this made a major contribution to developing my mental ability to concentrate and focus. I had to supply the motivation, desire to succeed and hard work but the intense brain exercise of competing in college in a language with an entirely new alphabet strengthened my mental capabilities. It's a long way from barely finishing high school to completing my medical training and receiving board certification in both psychiatry and neurology.

I am sure that my personal experiences helped me to develop successful and effective methods of treating adolescents with psychological difficulties many of whom showed clear ADHD symptoms. Raising three boys, one with similar symptoms of ADHD, gave me practical experience on a daily basis.

As a young psychiatrist and neurologist, I treated a large

number of adolescents and adults addicted to drugs and/or alcohol. Many had ADHD as well. With the treatment methods for alcohol and drug abuse in current use at that time, there was a "revolving door" phenomenon; patients went through treatment in a specialty hospitals or units for 30 to 90 days removed from their every day stresses at home and at work for intense therapy. Patients would return to their environment expressing that they were "reformed" and determined to remain sober. After a few months or a year or so, they would be back in treatment again. Adolescents were the same. They were determined to stay off drugs but far too many returned. There was a high degree of treatment failure. I developed a theory that it was the stresses in life and a breakdown in coping mechanisms that led to the abuse of alcohol and drugs. I believed the alcoholic needed to return to his environment as soon as possible and to be taught coping mechanisms and problem solving techniques while surrounded by the elements that caused the stress. The goal was to help the alcoholic to deal with the stresses that overwhelmed his coping mechanisms rather than to remove him to an unrealistic stress-free environment.

Since in 1980 this new approach contradicted the traditional approach, I had to find a partner who would be willing to support this new approach to treatment. Lockheed Georgia (now Lockheed-Martin), the largest industrial employer in Georgia at the time with about 30,000 employees agreed to sponsor this new treatment approach. In 1980 I founded and was medical director of the Advanced Recovery Center (ARC). This was the first day hospital in the U.S. for treatment of chemical dependency that was approved by the National Association of Hospitals. Today this form of treatment is the standard in the U. S. and many other countries as well.

Seeing hundreds of adolescents and adults at ARC, it became clear that between 25–35% of those who came for therapy had ADHD symptoms. These patients had to literally be taught new ways of thinking. From living for years without diagnosis or treatment, often they had poor self-esteem, no organizational skills, low academic achievements and a lack of direction in life. It was foolish to treat the alcohol or drug abuse without treating the underlying stresses.

My years as co-director of the marriage and sex counseling clinic at Emory Medical School department of Psychiatry revealed to me the turmoil ADHD causes in relationships with spouse and children. It was clearly a major cause of marital distress.

Analyzing the different treatment methods for ADHD led me to the conclusion that there ought to be a multi-disciplinary approach based on the most recent findings from the finest research centers. The best treatment has to involve daily mental and physical exercises. Aerobic exercise is the foundation for a healthy body but today we know that it also improves mental development and emotional stability. Teaching parents to coach their ADHD child every day and to empower the parents to take charge of the treatment effort is so much more effective than hoping for a 'quick fix' with Ritalin. Why not use the power of communication and every day conversations with your child to improve his thinking skills? Parents are in the best position to use crises, successes and failures, strengths and weaknesses to teach the thinking skills crucial to the growth and maturation of their child. Professionals can always be consulted to guide, assist, train, teach and provide any needed professional advice, but the main influence should be the parents.

The next step was to put these theories into practice and compare results with the work of leading research centers for confirmation. This led to the writing of this book.

There are treatment strategies across the life span from childhood through adolescence and adult stages in life. Of course, it is more complex if your teen is diagnosed with ADHD and has had no previous therapeutic intervention. More than likely, he has developed poor habits of organization, perhaps weak social skills or an unimpressive academic record and abysmal self esteem. It is very important to get your teen's ADHD symptoms under control quickly because this is a risky stage in life.

For example, driving can be very dangerous because of poor judgment, impulsivity and loss of concentration. Society expects more with each year of age and your teen may be immature in relation to his peers. Poor social skills and repeated academic failure often lead to joining marginal groups where he feels accepted.

ADHD symptoms often are expressed in different behavior in adults than in children. Obviously adults have developed many compensatory mechanisms that can be more or less effective. But if you look at negative behavior and feelings and compare employed adults with and without ADHD, you see the following:

	With ADHD to without ADHD
Addicted to tobacco	64 to 36%
Excessive use of alcohol	34 to 28%
Recreational drug use	52 to 33%
Been arrested	37 to 18%
Job changes in ten years	5.4 to 3.4
Divorced	28 to 15%
Good relationship with parents	47% to 70%
Fits in well with peers	40% to 70%

Those *Dissatisfied* with the following key aspects of life:

	With ADHD to without ADHD
Family life	68 to 47%
Relationship with partners	58 to 47%
Social Life	58 to 38%
Health and fitness	39 to 23%

Professional life	40 to 22%
Often feel sad and depressed	29 to 7%
Often act without thinking of the consequences	27 to 11%
Have a bright outlook on my future	40 to 67%

It cannot be emphasized enough that ADHD can be overcome. You should approach this challenge with a positive attitude. You face many challenges in life. This is one that, with persistence and patience, can be overcome.

Chapter 1

FACTS AND FICTION

There are so many myths and so much misinformation out there about ADHD that I want to set the record straight from the beginning. It is a real condition affecting about 10% of children. In just the last few years we have learned that there is a deficiency of neurotransmitter in the ADHD brain. This is where the problem is as well as the solution. It is not some imagined condition.

Ritalin is not addictive. It corrects the neurological deficit in about 70% of cases but the changes are not permanent. When medication is stopped, the symptoms return. For Ritalin to diminish the child's height, it would need to be taken every day for at least two years. Research suggests that when the medication is stopped, growth returns to normal levels. Ritalin is cleared from the body in about 4 hours. It is highly unlikely that Ritalin has any influence one way or the other on creativity, talent, etc.

Vigorous mental and physical exercises designed to stimulate neuronal growth and develop more sophisticated problem solving skills can correct the deficiency in neurotransmitter that is the cause of ADHD and eliminate the need for medication.

This is the first major improvement in the treatment of ADHD since Ritalin was developed 40 years ago.

Many famous people have had great success in life without intervention. Included among them are actors such as Will Smith, Sylvester Stallone, Jim Carey and Dustin Hoffman, athletes including Bruce Jenner and Magic Johnson, statesmen such as John and Robert Kennedy as well as entrepreneurs such as Charles Schwab. Clearly, ADHD does not preclude success in life. There is a small percentage of children with ADHD whom as adults are at the top of their field without treatment. ADHD does not preclude genius, creativity, talent, motivation, enthusiasm or charisma. Even though it is inspiring to be aware that we know of many successful individuals with ADHD, it is hard to imagine that the majority of these children will reach their full potential without diagnosis and treatment. There can be serious consequences to leaving ADHD untreated.

ADHD is so prevalent that many feel it to be a natural variant within the human species. This may be true. However, society has changed drastically over the last hundred years. In an agrarian society, perhaps being unable to study, read and concentrate for long periods of time was not such a terrible handicap. No one was driving a vehicle at 60mi/hr. Social relationships and professional demands were not as sophisticated as they are today. Today, a child or adult who is unable to focus, unable to control emotional outbursts or does not reflect on past mistakes, will have great difficulty in the complex world we live in today. This could explain why the "sudden" increase in cases of ADHD; it simply was not such a big problem in simpler times. *Society changed but biology did not.* Whatever the reason, it is foolish to be in denial and just hope for the best.

Poor academic performance, increased accidents, risky behavior and poor social skills as well as not fully utilizing information from past mistakes clearly have serious consequences. The goal is to move your child into the category that would be defined as a success story by any casual observer. So let's get started.

We understand the cause of ADHD at the cellular level. The

prefrontal lobe of the brain right behind the forehead is the part of the brain that controls higher more sophisticated thought processes. This is the part of the brain that makes man such a unique species. Relating the past and future, planning, making choices, controlling emotions are some of the functions of the frontal lobe. Weak neuronal transmissions in this critical part of the brain are the cause of ADHD. Impulsivity, difficulty with planning, poor working memory, inadequate problem solving skills and hyperactivity can now be positively and dramatically influenced by brain exercises. Every day experiences and challenges can be turned into mental exercises by parents who have acquired the skills to implement a training program for their children. Teaching these exercises is the main focus of this book.

ADHD is a conduction deficit at the neuronal synapse (a synapse is a microscopic space between two neurons critical to nerve conduction and transmission of information). If the conduction of an *inhibitory* impulse is weak, when the child has an urge to dart into the street, wander away from his mother or he wants to hit someone, he will do so without ever going through the inhibitory steps of considering the consequences. If the conduction is a *stimulatory* impulse and it is weak, the child (or adult) will show signs of inattention, forgetfulness and an inability to focus.

All mental activities need either neural stimulation or inhibition. If you think of the incidents where your ADHD child has difficulties, you will see that it is mainly a problem of weak inhibition or weak stimulation.

There has never been a time for such optimism. You should approach this learning experience with confidence, motivation and enthusiasm. Success is within your grasp.

▶ **WHAT IS THE PERSPECTIVE OF THOSE INVOLVED WITH ADHD?**

Children with ADHD hear disapproval on a daily basis from

both family and teachers. These children don't feel good about themselves because they constantly fail to meet the expectations of people who are important to them. All have a great deal more anxiety and frustration than most of their peers. While it is not a problem to play hours of video games, completing a few math problems in a homework assignment, paying attention to the teacher or reading detailed instructions are often doomed to failure. An inordinate amount of time is often spent searching for a misplaced backpack, homework and an assortment of other belongings. Activities of daily living, such as getting dressed also take much more time than needed. Often they seem oblivious and even cavalier about their behavior and find themselves more involved in day dreaming than problem solving. It is not unusual for these children to avoid confrontations by conveniently forgetting to bring home schoolbooks or homework assignments. If the subject is boring to the child, they will resort to procrastination or throwing tantrums because the demands placed on him exceed his ability to concentrate and focus.

From the perspective of the parent, there is obvious concern for their child's future. Often parents blame each other, the teacher or the system for the child's shortcomings. Feelings of shame and embarrassment can result from the child's behavior and complaints from school. Many are simply at a loss as to how to proceed. If parents compare their ADHD child to other children without ADHD, they realize they have a very high maintenance child who will argue over the simplest request such as getting up in the morning and going to bed at night, and often they feel they are in an ongoing power struggle over every issue. An ADHD child argues and fights to get what he wants and has the endurance to wear most parents down. He has the stamina and an arsenal of excuses for not going to bed, not doing his chores, not doing homework, etc. at the prescribed time and can push their parents to exhaustion and ultimately acquiescence.

From the perspective of the teacher, an ADHD child requires

an excessive amount of time and energy. The routine of the classroom is constantly being disrupted and the progress of the whole class is compromised. She observes a child with problems in the areas of focus, listening, hyperactivity and immaturity.

From the perspective of the clinician, ADHD is a medical condition that needs to be correctly diagnosed and treated. Usually, treatment involves Ritalin to alleviate the symptoms.

From the perspective of the scientist, ADHD is a mild neurological condition usually caused by hereditary factors (in about 80% of the cases). There are specific genes that cause changes at the synapse that weaken conductivity in the front part of the brain whose role is higher executive functions such as planning, impulse control, decision making, concentration, focus, emotions, etc.

From my perspective, an ADHD child or adult has many positive traits and capabilities but he will have cognitive deficiencies that cause him social, academic and emotional difficulties. The good new is that these deficiencies are surmountable.

▶ **NO NEED FOR DISTRESS IF YOUR CHILD HAS ADHD:**
Creating an environment with warm, consistent and unconditional love is the foundation for the ADHD child. If you are not a demonstrative person or have difficulty verbally expressing love and praise, get over it now. Even if it sounds "artificial" or not the "real you," make the effort. The more you practice, the easier and more natural it will become.

Raising three boys, one with symptoms of ADHD as early as age 4, gave me ongoing daily experience with this condition. In most children, these symptoms disappear by grade school.

However, when it was time to enter grade school, we decided to hold him back a year until he was more mature and ready to settle down. It was clear to us that there was no way he would be able to sit still as required. We searched for a school with small classes and lots of individual attention. Our strategy of holding him back a year did not solve the problem.

Things went pretty well in first grade as far as complaints from teachers about hyperactivity. However, he was diagnosed with a learning disability. In his case, he knew the alphabet and knew the sounds of the letters, but when he put them together in words, the words had no relationship to the sounds. We immediately began a reading program to focus on this weakness. The hyperactivity and lack of concentration together with a learning disability meant we had two completely separate problems, each of which required its own treatment.

We could tell our son was trying. Once he traced the outline of his feet on the floor under his desk to try to keep still and behave. More than once he came home very unhappy because the teacher was so upset with him. It definitely bothered him, but his "motor" was always running. We spent a great deal of time in parent-teacher conferences. I still remember his third grade teacher saying, "I feel like I spend half my time with your son and spread the other half among the rest of the class." We tried to channel all his excess energy into sports, where he excelled. Problems at school continued through good teachers and those who were not so good. I clearly remember when discussing the problems with one particular teacher. Her response to my comment that I thought, despite all the problems, our son was going to grow up to be just fine.

She ominously replied, "I'm not so sure." Forget teachers like that. Listen to those that tell you: "He has a heart of gold." "He's trying." "He's very kind." "We will keep trying." "He's a leader in his class."

I feel one of the reasons for his success as a young adult was because we focused on his strengths and talents and made sure he knew how much he was loved and how important he was to us. We initiated after school activities that were very helpful without realizing they contributed to reducing his ADHD symptoms. He took piano lessons every week. He hated practicing, but with praise and encouragement, he continued for many years. Now that we understand the etiology of ADHD, it is easy to see why this was also therapeutic. He played every sport possible. Later in college and after, instead of avoiding reading, he took on scholarly endeavors that involved a great deal of concentration such as the study of Talmudic law. (Find a subject that your child is passionate about and then get him lots of books on the topic). Of course, this also was excellent treatment for his learning disability as well as addressing the deficiency in synaptic neurotransmitters. Later, he developed proficiency in two other languages, some of the best training possible for brain stimulation and growth.

ADHD also reared its head in the fourth generation of my family. One of our nine grandchildren has classic ADHD symptoms. I feel very fortunate that therapeutic techniques without medication are available to this wonderful child today.

► **CAN POOR PARENTING CAUSE ADHD?**

No. The role of parents is perhaps the single most misunderstood aspect of ADHD. There is a tremendous amount of outdated and incorrect information about the causes of ADHD. As a result, parents tend to blame themselves or others for their child's condition. Often, guilt-ridden parents ask, "Where did we do wrong?" Other times, the parents may be criticized for not being sufficiently strict or attentive. In many cases, parents even blame one another. They may blame each other for somehow causing or exacerbating the child's condition. Poor parenting cannot cause ADHD, but certainly stress in the family such as divorce or separation or an unhappy home can cause ADHD-*like* symptoms. I emphasize learning how to be *effective* parents; most parents want the best for their child.

One father expressed remorse at not understanding his son for so many years. All those years he thought his son was lazy or spoiled or maybe slow. His attitude toward his son affected much of his young life. Only as a teenager was the boy diagnosed with ADHD – only then did he understand that his son suffered from a biological problem, and not a behavioral one.

► **WHAT FACTORS ARE INVOLVED IN ADHD?**

The causes of ADHD can be divided into two groups: genetic and non-genetic.

1. Genetic Causes of ADHD

Recent studies have shown that ADHD has a high level of inheritability. About 80% of cases of ADHD are inherited.

- Close to 40% of children with ADHD have a mother or father with ADHD.
- Siblings of children with ADHD have a 50% higher probability of being diagnosed with the same condition.
- Studies done on [identical] twins that were raised in different families have shown a high degree of similar symptoms, regardless of their home environment.
- Studies done over the past 30 years show that ADHD is present across all ethnic groups around the world.

Like height or blue eyes, it appears ADHD is biologically inherited.

2. Non-Genetic Causes of ADHD

Except for injury to the front part of the brain, there are only a few known non-genetic causes of ADHD.

A. Gestational Factors:

– Twenty-two percent of mothers who smoked during pregnancy will have an ADHD child, as compared with 8% of non-smoking mothers.

– Alcohol exposure during pregnancy causes an increased incidence of ADHD.

– Low birth weight is another factor linked to ADHD, as well as complications in pregnancy and delivery.

– Birth injury

B. Psychological Adversity:

Maternal psychopathology can be a major factor in the development of ADHD-like symptoms. Children with a clinically depressed parent have a two to three-fold increase in ADHD-like symptoms. Further, it has been shown that 25% of children with ADHD and conduct disorders will have a mother or father with a conduct disorder.

Major family conflict (separation, divorce, on-going conflict in the home between the mother and father), low social class, or the removal of a child from his home, were all found to be associated with ADHD-like symptoms in children.

C. Modern technology:

Our brains are massively remodeled by exposure to the Internet – but it's also remodeled by reading, television, video games, electronics, music, and more. These devices can be powerful tools for good and for bad.

In a recent study of 2600 toddlers between the ages of one and three, watching television correlated with impulse and attention problems later in childhood. For every hour of TV watched per day, the probability that they would develop serious attention deficits at the age of seven increased by 10%. The study did not rule out other possible contributors. It might be that children with attention deficits are more often put in front of the TV by their parents, but it is suggestive and a cause for concern. It is wise to severely limit TV before the age of three, if at all. Harvard psychiatrist, Edward Hallowell, an ADD expert, has linked the electronic media to the rise of attention deficit.

Head injury:

It is astonishing how many completely forget or do not mention a serious head trauma that occurred in early childhood.

Is it justified to blame yourself for your child's symptoms?
Focus should remain on constructive steps that can be taken to help the child. Parents, educators and caregivers can collaborate with an ADHD child and each other to bring about positive change and improved functioning. Don't blame yourself.

▶ **CAN A CREATIVE, SOCIABLE, SMART CHILD HAVE ADHD?**

Another example of ADHD symptoms is described by the following episode:

Mrs. Parker, Miriam's mother, came to the clinic to evaluate her daughter's emotional state. Miriam's mother describes her as creative, sociable and smart. What caused the family constant stress was her moodiness. She was easily angered, argumentative and defiant over activities of daily living that meant a daily confrontation over many different issues. It was quite common for Miriam to wake up in the bad mood and often bedwetting was an issue. Then there's a daily struggle about brushing her hair or getting dressed or fighting with siblings. The slightest frustration can result in a tantrum or excessive crying. Although Miriam is only 7 years old, she already has a reputation in school as a smart girl who is quite disorganized, frequently loses papers, pencils and other belongings and is unable to sustain attention. The result is continuously making careless mistake, failure to finish tasks and performing below her intelligence and ability level. Miriam would be known as a chatterbox and when following her thinking, it is clear she has long drawn out answers that are not well thought through, disorganized or rambling. Assignments that should take no more than 30–45 minutes might take several hours. She is also distracted by every noise or activity around her that cause her to make careless mistakes or to abandon the task entirely.

A summary of Miriam's symptoms include:
- Restless
- Fidgets

- Disorganized
- Forgetful
- Difficulty sustaining attention
- Careless mistakes
- Fails to finish tasks
- Not listening
- Blurts out answers
- Talks excessively
- Easily distracted
- Constant power struggles
- Explosive behavior
- Repeats similar mistakes

▶ **SO HOW CAN THIS BE A "REAL" DISORDER WHEN MY CHILD CAN FOCUS AND CONCENTRATE FOR HOURS ON VIDEO GAMES, TV, SPORTS, ETC. WITH NO PROBLEM WHATSOEVER?**

This was very puzzling to parents. ADD manifests itself only in the "uninteresting" activities but is absent in "interesting" or exciting activities. The child can rivet his attention on anything he finds pleasurable. Attention drifts on any task without instant gratification such as homework. To parents and teachers, this often looked like laziness, immaturity or lack of motivation. The child can *not* perform the task he is facing because it has been demonstrated that neuronal activity actually *decreases* when concentration is needed for tasks. There is a center in the frontal lobe of the brain specifically concerned with goal-setting and delayed gratification but a malfunction in this region of the brain was not related to ADHD symptoms until recently.

This brain center must be strengthened. *No amount of punishment or discipline will cause the formation of the deficient neurotransmitters.*

► **IMPORTANT POINTS TO REMEMBER:**

- ADHD is a biological genetic condition in the brain in 80% of cases.
- ADHD is caused be a weakness in the synapse that causes weak conductivity.
- ADHD children can reach their potential.
- There are techniques for building a stronger, more flexible and quicker brain.
- Several signs should alert parents to possible ADHD symptoms.
- Most children with ADHD will show combined symptoms of hyperactivity and inattention.
- Among those with ADHD, a group of about 27% will show inattention only.
- We will treat the *cause* of ADHD instead of treating the symptoms.

Chapter 2

THE HISTORY AND DIAGNOSIS OF ADHD

Though some may think of ADHD as the latest "en vogue" diagnosis, it is actually not a new condition. Dr. George Still in 1902 gave a series of lectures to the Royal College of Physicians in London where he described the syndrome in terms very similar to the way we see it today. He described these children as having "inhibition of the will"- an inability to control themselves or function effectively in group activities. He also reported later that these traits ran in families and that the mothers of these children were more likely to be depressed.

In 1937 Charles Bradley reported his findings in the American Journal of Psychiatry. In this study he reported improvement in concentration and reduced hyperactivity in children with similar symptoms after treatment with Benzadrine. At the time, Benzadrine was sold in the U.S. as over the counter treatment for allergies, upper respiratory complaints and headaches. Dr. Bradley used Benzadrine to treat children with ADHD symptoms who also complained of severe headaches. The sudden improvement in the children's concentration was unexpected and surprising to doctors. From that point on, the Bradley Children's Home in Rhode Island gave the children with ADHD symptoms Benzedrine and observed that they performed better in math after receiving the medication.

In 1955 methylphenidate (Ritalin) was developed as a new medication to help children with similar symptoms. Both Benzedrine and methylphenidate (Ritalin) belong to the class of drugs known as central nervous system stimulants. Doctors are often like detectives. They must identify symptoms (clues) and try to discover the cause (culprit).

In the mid 1960s, Sam Clements pointed out for the first time that the inability to sustain attention was the main symptom of this condition in otherwise healthy children. Up until that time, hyperactivity symptoms had been the main focus of this unnamed condition. Some with ADHD have hyperactivity but all have attention deficits.

▶ **HOW CAN YOU TELL IF YOUR CHILD HAS ADHD?**

Most of the clinics around the world are using criteria developed and published by the American Psychiatric Association in their official publications. To diagnose ADHD, certain conditions or symptoms need to be present in three areas of general functioning:

A. Inattention that is not age appropriate:
- Makes frequent careless mistakes and doesn't cope well with details
- Has difficulty sustaining attention when reading, playing or doing homework
- Poor listening skills
- Poorly organizational skills
- Fails to follow instructions
- Fails to finish tasks such as homework and chores
- Avoids tasks that require sustained concentration such as reading, homework

- Constantly loses possessions
- Distracted easily by minor outside stimuli, such as music, voices or noise
- Forgetful

B. Impulsivity:
- Blurts out answers before questions are completed
- Fails to wait his turn in games or other activities
- Often interrupts or intrudes on others and displays aggression
- Emotional outbursts that are not age appropriate
- Little or no frustration tolerance

C. Hyperactivity:
- Unable to sit still
- Unusual restlessness
- Fidgety
- Always "on the go"
- Talks incessantly
- Difficulty playing quiet games

▶ **CONDITIONS THAT NEED TO BE PRESENT FOR A DIAGNOSIS OF ADHD:**

Although many children will present different symptoms initially, *all* children diagnosed with ADHD have to fulfill all the following criteria:

1. At least six symptoms from the Inattention domain
2. Six symptoms taken from either the Impulsivity or Hyperactivity domain or both
3. Symptoms must have been present for at least six months
4. Some of the symptoms must have been present before 7 years of age
5. Some of the impairment from symptoms must be present in two settings such as home and school

6. Symptoms must have led to significant impairment in social or academic functioning

Therefore, information is critical from parents, teachers and other school professionals or caregivers. To make a diagnosis of ADHD, the above criteria must be met. Sometimes other medical diagnostic tests such as blood tests, neuro-imaging, x-ray, electro-encephalogram (EEG) are performed to rule out other medical conditions that may have some of the same symptoms. These tests are not routinely performed, but may be needed in a few cases. It is important to remember that all children have ADHD-type symptoms to some degree at some points in their lives. However, classic ADHD children suffer from these symptoms to the extent that they are *unable* to perform up to their intellectual ability and are *impaired* in their expected emotional development.

There will be a variation in the symptoms in terms of severity, frequency and pervasiveness in each child and symptoms may change in different settings and may vary in the same setting at different times. We must observe and evaluate how the child is functioning in different environments and in multiple settings on different days in order to see the overall areas of life where the child is experiencing greater than normal difficulties with activities of daily living and learning. In a few children, severe problems may not present until high school when academic demands are more challenging because their charm or intelligence has allowed them to fly under the radar.

Although we have established clear symptoms and criteria to diagnose ADHD, a definitive diagnosis is often difficult to make. Many of the symptoms and criteria are subjective and there is no objective way to define them or test for them. Some medical tests can rule out other medical conditions and psychological testing can determine possible learning disabilities or identify some specific area of concern in the emotional and developmental stages of a child, but they are not diagnostic for ADHD.

Today the diagnosis of ADHD is based on clinical history.

Therefore, it is absolutely necessary to gather information from as many sources as possible, including parents, caregivers, teachers and other professional staff who have had contact with the child. It is not unusual to receive conflicting history from each parent or from parents and teachers or parents and caregivers. Remember there must be symptoms in *more* than one environment. A child whose behavior is normal at home but out of control at school or vice versa; that child does not have ADHD. Only after receiving information from all significant sources and the elimination of other issues such as allergies, excessive stress in the home, sleep disorders, seizure disorders, etc. can a definitive diagnosis be made.

► **USE OF RATING SCALE:**

The use of a rating scale to assess ADHD is quite helpful. A rating scale helps establish the developmental level of a child in comparison with established norms. It helps in screening for specific symptoms that can point out the existence of other conditions such as learning disabilities and help to clarify the differential diagnosis. In elementary schools, the more popular rating scales used in the process of diagnosis is the Child Behavioral Check List (CBCL). Conner's Parents and Teachers Rating Scales is the most comprehensive and reliable for children age 3 to 17. It allows us to look at eight categories:
- Oppositional behavior
- Cognitive problems
- Hyperactivity/ impulsive behavior
- Anxiety-shyness
- Perfectionism
- Social problems
- Psychosomatic complaints
- DSM IV symptoms, subscales and ADHD Index. (see definition in footnotes).

The Teacher Rating Scales contain 59 items that parallel the

Parenting Rating Scale. These scales provide baseline observations to which the child's progress will be compared. Repeating this rating scale will allow monitoring of the child's progress over a treatment period.

▶ **USE OF NEUROPSYCHOLOGICAL TESTS:**

Neuropsychological tests are not diagnostic, but may be useful. They should be used to rule out other diagnoses.

▶ **TEST OF VARIABLES OF ATTENTION:**

TOVA is a computerized assessment procedure in which a visual continuous performance test (CPT) is conducted for 25 minutes. The child presses a firing button whenever a correct target stimulus is present on the screen of the computer. The same test is repeated after the child is given a single dose of Ritalin and the responses are compared. If the results are significantly better after the medication, taking into account that the child is now more familiar with the test, the improved results are attributed to Ritalin. This procedure is non-language based to differentiate ADD from learning disorders and require no right-left discrimination. *The most glaring problem with* TOVA *is the high number of false positives that indicate there are attention deficits, even when ADHD is not present. This test is not endorsed in the American Academy of Pediatrics guidelines for diagnosis of ADHD and it is not in common clinical use in the U.S. and many other countries.*

▶ **OTHER MEDICAL CONDITIONS TO BE RULED OUT:**

We must give consideration to other medical conditions that may present similar symptoms. Sleep disturbances impact some children, causing symptoms similar to ADHD. Seizures or thyroid problems could also result in similar symptoms.

Lead poisoning will cause ADHD-like symptoms. Allergies can produce ADHD-like symptoms.

Developmental disorders such as autism, non-verbal learning

disabilities and Asperger's Syndrome should be ruled out. Tic disorder as well as psychotic conditions such as manic depressive states need to be ruled out. Head trauma, especially any injury to the frontal lobe or cerebellum, needs to be evaluated. It is amazing how often I find that serious accidents are not mentioned in a typical interview.

▶ **PSYCHOLOGICAL FACTORS:**

Divorce or separation of parents can bring about severe reactions in a child. Many situations in the family such as loss of a job, illness, neglect as well as mental, physical or sexual abuse can all contribute to symptoms similar to ADHD in a child.

▶ **CO-EXISTING CONDITIONS:**

An array of co-existing conditions may complicate the diagnosis and treatment of ADHD. They may include learning disabilities, oppositional behavior, anxiety and depression.

▶ **IMPORTANT POINTS TO REMEMBER:**
- Every child must have a thorough physical and neurological examination to determine that they are generally healthy. As long as the neurological system is healthy, there is no need for extensive neurological tests and procedures.
- Before medication is prescribed, a physical examination should eliminate any cardiovascular anomalies.
- Complete rating scales by parents and teachers are an essential part of the evaluation.
- Diagnosis of ADHD is based on the confirmation of at least six symptoms of inattention and six symptoms of impulsivity and hyperactivity for a total of twelve. These symptoms need to be present both at home *and* at school for at least six months.
- Family stress can cause ADHD-like symptoms.
- Symptoms must cause impairment of functioning in the life of the child.

- Some of the symptoms must start before the age of seven.
- Psychological testing can be useful in identifying learning disabilities or specific areas of weakness, but it is not diagnostic.
- The diagnosis of ADHD can only be made by a compilation of history and information obtained by family, teachers and the child.
- ADHD frequently persists from childhood to adolescence and throughout adulthood and will adversely impact development across the lifespan.
- The child with ADHD will show symptoms when he is bored or uninterested in the task at hand. The symptoms of inability to focus will be less than predicted for his age.
- Because ADHD children have a poor working memory, they may be afraid they will forget an answer and will therefore blurt one out as quickly as possible.
- Being impulsive means that these children will not exhibit caution at appropriate times. They may dart into the street or suddenly be in dangerous circumstances when the parent is distracted for only a moment. Parents need to keep this in mind.

Chapter 3

PARENTS AND FAMILY

► **THE IMPORTANT ROLE OF PARENTS:**

Although a vast number of ADHD cases have biological origins, the role of family in helping the ADHD child is of the utmost importance. Evidence suggests that children with ADHD who receive treatment experience improved outcome in social, academic and later occupational spheres of their lives. Effective help administered as early as possible will lower the risk for developing many of the mental health problems ranging from low self-esteem to conduct disorders that are prevalent in individuals with ADHD.

Proper medication, combined with effective physical exercise and cognitive development, lowers the severity and frequency of inattention and hyperactivity in an ADHD child. Medication does not produce permanent changes in the brain, but it does give parents the opportunity to initiate brain exercises in a calmer more focused child. Despite the demonstrated efficacy of medication, evidence suggests that adherence to a medication regime is disappointingly low. Within 12 months of follow up, adherence rate for medication averaged about 20%. It is easy to understand a parent's aversion to giving any medication to a young child every day.

A 2006 study showed a correlation between the number of office visits and a child's adherence to medication. This suggests that the opportunity to meet with clinicians and discuss ADHD symptoms and problems, as well as to ask for direction and advice, is effective in improving adherence to medical treatment. Since parents are the most consistent people in a child's life and are committed to his well-being, their role in the treatment process is central and critical. Parents can coach, encourage and motivate their child better than anyone else to overcome his symptoms and gain mastery over his behavior. It cannot be emphasized enough how important parental influence is for a successful outcome as a child struggles to overcome his handicaps.

► **WHAT IS THE IMPACT OF THE ADHD CHILD ON A FAMILY?**

All of us have weaknesses or handicaps of one kind or another. In this instance, it is not only possible, but imperative to empower parents and help them develop the skills that will enable them to coach their children in successful life skills. The parent-child and sibling-child interaction in a family of a child with ADHD have been shown to be more negative and stressful for all family members than typical interactions in families when ADHD is not present.

The ADHD child has a major impact on his family by creating constant stress through excessive and unreasonable demands, inconsistent behavior and constant need for inordinate attention that can destabilize the family routine and atmosphere. The relentless stress and friction between all family members leads to higher divorce rates and other symptoms of family conflict.

► **WHAT IS THE IMPACT OF PARENTS ON AN ADHD CHILD?**

Mothers of children with ADHD spend an enormous amount of time trying to modify their child's behavior, resolve the chronic difficulties they face, and struggle with persistent issues of disorganization, inattention and inappropriate behavior. Needless to say, other family members may be neglected. Interestingly, the father, who usually spends less time with an ADHD child during the day, is often better able to elicit appropriate responses when interacting with the child. It may be that fathers tend to give firm and short commands that get the child's attention and as a result, the task is completed faster and with less conflict. It may also be that the child is more intimidated by his father. A child's varying response to each parent can increase stress between parents, with the father becoming critical of the mother's parenting and vice versa.

▶ **IMPACT ON OTHER SIBLINGS:**

It is quite natural to see children respond differently to mothers and fathers, especially children with ADHD. This may lead to frustration and negative feelings toward the child. In families with siblings, the situation can become quite complicated and difficult to manage. The most difficult relationship seems to be between two brothers with similar conditions. When an older brother or sister has ADHD, the younger siblings seem to have numerous adjustment difficulties. The nature of the siblings' interactions depends on their personalities and the relationship of the older brother or sister in the family with the parents. As long as the relationship between the older sibling with ADHD and the parents is good and stable, they serve as a shield to the younger sibling that encourages a better relationship between them.

▶ **REACTION OF SIBLING TO HIS ADHD BROTHER OR SISTER:**

Reactions of the siblings who live with an ADHD brother or sister can be quite different. Living in a disruptive situation where conflict and stress are chronic can lead to feelings of resentment and anger. A sibling may feel victimized or feel that their brother is consistently causing stress and conflict, or that the parents neglect them to deal with the more problematic child. Others will respond differently. They will feel a sense of responsibility and will try to help the parents manage their brother's condition. Others may feel trapped, anxious and wary. Well-trained and informed parents will be better able to minimize the negative impact on their family and help siblings understand and deal more effectively with their ADHD sibling.

▶ HOW DO PARENTS WITH ADHD IMPACT AN ADHD CHILD?

A large number of children with ADHD are born to parents with existing similar difficulties. Clearly a father who has ADHD that was never properly diagnosed or treated can have a major negative impact on the child and other family members. He may also be impulsive, short tempered, explosive and unable to deal with frustration. Only a very small percentage of adult ADHD has been diagnosed and treated. In such cases, if parents can not help their child, then another caretaker such as a grandparent or nanny needs to learn the necessary skills. However, the parents should try hard to take on this role by asking their doctor about taking medication and use brain exercises to develop more effective mental functioning. ADHD adults should commit to daily aerobic exercise.

Many mothers who experience depression are unable to effectively help their ADHD child. Depression for a mother with a child without ADHD could be considered a medical emergency. Clearly, expecting a depressed mother to nurture her ADHD child is unrealistic. A father whose own life is not stable will find it very difficult, if not impossible, to help his ADHD child as he often also has issues with self-esteem, low tolerance for frustration and inadequate emotional assets.

▶ **PARENTS WHO EXPERIENCE STRESS AND ITS IMPACT ON THEIR CHILD:**

Life can be full of many unrelated crises such as a medical emergency or financial distress, as well as unresolved issues within the parents' relationship. Caring adequately for an ADHD child has a very poor prognosis under these circumstances. Often the conflict of how to handle the child contributes to the decision to divorce or separate. Now the single parent family will be under even more stress as additional tasks and responsibilities and usually a lower financial base are thrust upon her. Without adequate support, effective intervention and proper coaching, the probability that the condition of the ADHD child will deteriorate is great. These disruptive influences as well as any other change in the stability and consistency of family life cause much more stress in children with ADHD.

▶ **FOUR TYPES OF PARENTING:**

We will compare Permissive, Authoritarian and Dictatorial Parenting Models to a new style of parenting: The Coaching Parent.

The Permissive Parent

Today many parents grant their children a great deal of freedom in the hopes that this style of parenting will allow them to grow and develop confidence and independence. They do set some limits, but frequently do not impose them. Sometimes it is hard for this type of parent to say no. When this style of parenting does not produce the desired results, the parent can become angry, lose control, scream at the child and switch to a more demanding style of parenting.

The Authoritarian Parent

The authoritarian parent has a rigid set of rules and regulations. The limits are quite clear and the tasks and expectations are expressed openly with clear consequences if the tasks are not completed. There are no gray areas. Everything is explained and the expectation is that the child will follow the rules and regulations. When the child does not respond as expected, the authoritarian parent loses his temper and uses different types of punishment to enforce the rules.

The Dictatorial Parent

Some parents act as dictators in their homes. The child usually does as he is told out of fear of consequences and the severe punishment he will receive. The impact of this style of parenting is that the child will never develop feelings of confidence and self esteem will be low. The child may develop dependency on other children or people. As an adolescent, they tend to join different types of marginal groups or street gangs.

The Coaching Parent

I would like to propose a different type of parenting that may be optimal for helping a child with ADHD: The Coaching Parent. To coach a child through the complexities of life, one must be very involved in the parenting process. The parent should be a model, teaching or coaching all the time. The child and the parent should be on same team, working together to accomplish clear goals.

These goals or targets are planned together and methods to accomplish them will be fully explained and discussed. Simple and clear steps are planned and often practiced several times so that each task will be successfully completed. Not so different from team sports, the coach sets the limits, rules and regulations that each team member is expected to follow. The coach as the leader of the team earns respect based on his capabilities to help the team win. The parent-coach may use other professionals to help his team get the best advice and insight. These experts should include teachers and other professional staff in the school, the physician that prescribes medication and other specialists depending on the specific needs of the child. In all cases, it is very important that the child perceive with confidence that everyone is on the same team. The parent-coach will acquire the knowledge and skills to help the child develop the skills he needs as well as to improve the understanding and cooperation of other siblings.

Just as a coach works to improve the skills of every member of his team, so too parents should inspire and encourage their child to practice and develop the social and emotional skills necessary for a happy constructive life. As with most efforts in life, practice and more practice is essential to improve or develop new skills. First the parent-coach must acquire knowledge about new methods and guidelines for coaching the ADHD child in the tasks of daily living and the demands and expectations that he will confront. If there are other weaknesses, such as a learning disability, this too must be tackled simultaneously as part of the treatment process.

► **IMPORTANT POINTS TO REMEMBER:**

- The role of the parents in the treatment of the ADHD child is central and critical in determining his future success.
- Disorganized and dysfunctional family life as a result of alcoholism, anti-social behavior, depression, medical problems, loss of a job, etc. can cause poor functioning parents. This, of course, leads to serious collateral damage in an ADHD child.
- The coaching parent style requires much more involvement in teaching, training and developing life skills to deal with challenges. Coaching is a term that includes purposeful and targeted Teaching, Nurturing and Training – as powerful as TNT!
- Adults with ADHD should commit to daily aerobic exercise as well as mental challenges.

Chapter 4

LEARN TO BECOME A COACHING PARENT

▶ **WHAT DOES IT TAKE TO BECOME A COACHING PARENT?**

This chapter will give you guidelines, understanding and advice in developing the skills necessary to become an excellent coach. Be positive. Do not even think of giving up! Children become happy, stable and very successful adults with the help of their loving patient parents. You'll need patience because you are embarking on a long term coaching process. The path to success is a plan of action and clear goals. As the leader in this effort, you must first take care of yourself and your needs. Just like the stewardess on the airplane before takeoff instructs parents who are flying with small children to first put the oxygen mask on themselves before putting one on the child, so too must mothers of an ADHD child take care of themselves first. You must have outlets that allow you to relax and enjoy your day, feel good about yourself and take pride in this effort and other aspects of your life. Under these circumstances, the time and effort devoted to your child's difficulties will not be overwhelming. It's a matter of balance and if the mother is not happy, it is impossible to imagine that she can be involved in effective coaching.

▶ **BASIC RULES FOR BECOMING A GOOD COACH AS A PARENT:**

Most people will admit that parenting is the most difficult job they have experienced. Raising a child is the most important task parents will face and the one for which they have the least guidance or training. Loving and caring for your child is not enough; you must know how to show it. For example, if parents do not set clear boundaries for children, this is often interpreted by the child as a lack of love, even though the parent may perceive it differently. Putting money aside for a child's education is a sign of love but not one a small child can relate to. If you are not a demonstrative person, *change your behavior.* Efforts should be made to express praise as often as possible. Praise for achievements or completed tasks as well as *consistent* expressions of love and a positive attitude will form the foundation for developing confidence and self-esteem in a young child. It has been shown that parents say nine negative statements to their child for every one of praise. Reverse this order.

To develop a sense of stability in the house and comfort for the child, you must be *decisive, believe in yourself and be consistent.* Do not doubt that what you are asking of your child is reasonable and do not be hesitant in your insistence that he assume responsibilities and complete a given task. It is quite likely that you will make mistakes from time to time. This is normal and your expressed love for your child will compensate for any possible mistake. Your ADHD child is looking for parental leadership. You will begin to gain respect and appreciation when you are a strong leader whose actions and decisions are consistent. When met with defiance, never give in or you will get more of the same defiant behavior in the future. In fact, a child will push his boundaries until your limits are reached because often he has been able to get away with defiant behavior. Don't forget, children are masters of manipulation, and you are their testing ground for what works and what doesn't work. Do not change your realistic expectations about your child's behavior.

▶ **LEARN TO GIVE EFFECTIVE INSTRUCTIONS:**

As a parent-coach, it is up to you to show decisiveness in your expectations. If you were a coach of a basketball team, it would be totally unacceptable for a player to challenge your game plan and refuse to follow instructions. As your child's coach (and with full knowledge that everyone in the family is on the same team and must pull together in order to be successful) all your instructions should be presented with full anticipation that they will be carried out. Present your instructions in a firm voice and a matter-of-fact style. For example: "Take your school bag from the living room and put it in your room, please." "Clean up your room before going out to play, please". Do not start the request with: "I think you should" or" I would be happy if…"

Another effective form of instruction includes two parts: Combine a directive with a reward. "You can go to your friend's house after cleaning your room" "You can go outside and play as soon as you finish your homework." A young child will frequently challenge your instructions, especially in the beginning. Challenges from a child may take the form of "why do I have to do it" or "I will do it later." You need to keep your response short and direct. "Because I said so" is a short, simple and underused statement that does not require an explanation or negotiations. Once you have made your decision and you state it, maintain this position. In order to eliminate unnecessary conflict, you should think about your request and feel confident it is appropriate. Do not allow your leadership position to be challenged and do not acquiesce.

► **FIRST TASK OF THE COACHING PARENT:**

Among the early objectives, a parent-coach needs to establish in the home a set of rules, regulations and limits. There should be clear boundaries that are not negotiable. These rules should be discussed with the child to confirm they are fully understood. As the child matures, of course the rules will be modified to be age appropriate. The younger the child is, the simpler the rules should be. It is a good idea to have the rules written and a copy posted in the kitchen, in the playroom and in the child's room as a constant reminder. It also keeps the child focused on a time table of events during the day. These rules need to be agreed upon between the parents before it is presented to the child to completely eliminate undermining each other.

► **SPIRIT OF WINNING:**

Before we continue learning how to become an effective parent-coach and clearly defining the responsibilities of the "coaching staff," I'd like to share a pep talk given to my college football team by our coach. The coach was a realistic man with high expectations for our team. Before our summer training season, he would give a short speech:

"We're going to have a great season this year," he said, "and I'm setting three goals for the team. Number one: Win! Number two: Win! Number three: Win!

I hope that's clear. But as much as I do love winning, I'm also a practical man. During the off season the staff attended seminars on improving our teaching skills. I know we too can be more effective as a team. I know your strengths and weaknesses…we're going to capitalize on your strengths. Each of you will be placed in a position to maximize your potential. The season in front of us will be challenging. It will require that each of us do our best, despite conflicting schedules and responsibilities, whether it be exams or a part-time job. But if you don't commit to putting in work and effort on the field, we will fail. I know we may not win every game, but we must put forth our best effort to try and win each and every one. After each game, we will analyze the results so we can learn from our mistakes and improve our performance. With maximum effort you can expect maximum success. And in the end, you'll be proud of what you've accomplished."

► **BE THE HEAD COACH OF YOUR TEAM:**

The parent who spends the most time with the child must assume the role of "head coach." The other parent must be on an equal footing concerning responsibilities and decision-making. You must unify the 'coaching staff' at home which includes the mother, father and any other adults or mature children. If grandparents or a caregiver has a regular role in caring for your child, they must understand how they can be helpful and what they need to do.

You must speak the same language, understand each other, set common goals and decide on a plan of action and methods to help the child. These are not simple goals for parents but you must reach common ground to work as a team. Without this unified effort, the attempts to help the child will fail. Just like the coaching staff of a college football team, parents must recognize and appreciate their child's strengths and weaknesses. Most ADHD children have strengths that are often not recognized or in some cases ignored. You must look for and identify areas of strength in your child because these will be powerful tools in your child's development.

► **LEARN TO STATE YOUR INSTRUCTIONS:**

As an effective parent-coach your instructions and directions have to be:
- Short
- Simple
- Clear – Without room for interpretation

For example, during a visit to a playground or to any other fun activity, most ADHD children will not respond well to statements like "It's time to go." Because ADHD children have difficulty switching from one activity to another, you need to give your instructions in stages. For example, make sure that the child really hears you when you say, "In five minutes, we have to leave" or "When the show you are watching is over, we have to leave." Follow this with the question: "David, did you hear me?" If in doubt, you should ask: "Can you repeat what I just said?" After five minutes, you should state, "David, turn off the TV and put your coat on, we are leaving." With appropriate chores assigned to the child, it is more effective to say "You can play outside but first go to your room and put all the games on your table back on the book shelf and make your bed." In other words, don't give the general command "to clean your room." First put the positive – you can play and then very specific tasks, not just 'clean your room.' Homework is, of course, a major challenge for all ADHD children. This will be dealt with in detail later in the chapter.

▶ **IMPROVE YOUR FAMILY LIFE – SET A WEEKLY MEETING WITH YOUR TEAM:**

Since the behavior of ADHD children can be predicted, we need to develop plans to counteract misbehavior. Most parents react to their child's behavior on an emotional level without clear plans or goals. The results of these unplanned reactions lead to negative, unproductive interactions. Hostility and anger lead to feelings of helplessness, frustration and often despair. Remember the example of the football coach who has a weekly meeting with the team to discuss and plan for challenges of the next game. You have to do the same. Take proactive steps to prepare for the next confrontation. Sometimes you can tailor your approach to fit your child. If it is always difficult to get the homework assignment done, try breaking the task into shorter simpler parts to make it less overwhelming. For example, tell your child that after he finishes the first part of his homework assignment, he can take a break to play outside for 30 minutes. You have to find what makes a difficult chore easier for your child. Try to anticipate or predict the usual reaction of your child to a challenge. You can coach your child to respond to new and old challenges in more productive ways.

This weekly "coaching meeting" with your child will help build a better team effort as you tackle difficulties together, rather than as adversaries. You can view this in the same way as preparations for a long car trip. Surely you would devote time and effort to planning the trip in such as way as to maximize the benefits to you and your child. You would plan numerous stops, include entertainment and age appropriate activities along the way rather than just get in the car and drive for hours without stopping. If you do not plan and just drive straight through, the entire trip will be stressful and unproductive. You will get the job done, but the price will be very high and the purpose defeated. This model needs to be kept in mind when you face a problem or task that you want your child to complete.

▶ **THE NEED TO DEAL WITH ONE ISSUE AT A TIME:**

Choose one issue, task or goal that you want to achieve. Begin thinking and planning the steps to accomplish this goal. This principle should apply to routine tasks such as homework or chores as well as to more complex tasks such as social interactions or organizational skills. You want the goal to be completed in such a way that both of you feel good about the accomplishment. Keep in mind that the process of reaching the goal is as important as the goal itself. Completing the task in a productive peaceful atmosphere, without fights or arguments, will not only continue to improve the positive atmosphere at home, but will also strengthen your relationship with your child and above all, help to build self confidence – the key ingredient to success in life as an adult.

Never forget praise; it's emotional nourishment.

Why do ADHD children forget homework assignments?

The ADHD child has difficulties in two specific areas of memory:

1. His working memory is poor. (Adults who have forgotten where they parked their car at the mall can relate) This is one of the reasons they tend to blurt out answers or answer out of turn; they are afraid they will forget the answer.

2. Accessing past experiences is also lagging. ADHD children often seem to not learn from their mistakes. They make similar mistakes over and over. Either they do not encode the information the first time or they act so impulsively that reflecting on past mistakes never happens.

▶ HOW TO HELP YOUR CHILD DO HIS HOMEWORK:

Let's go through a typical confrontation over homework.

Mother to 8-year-old son: "Ben, I noticed that you spent several hours doing your homework yesterday but you did not finish it. Then you spent the rest of the evening being upset. What is going on?"

(The mother already has in her mind a plan to try to correct the situation).

Ben: "I hate doing homework."

Mother: "I know you hate doing homework."

Ben: "It's too hard for me and I do not understand some of it. Also it's too much."

Mother: "You are telling me that the homework is too hard and they give too much."

Ben: "Yes, way too much and too hard."

Mother: "Well, you know that homework is part of school and every child who goes to school needs to do his homework to be successful and advance to the next grade."

Ben: I don't have to."

Mother: "This is a problem we can work on together and solve. Let's think about it together."

Ben: "How?"

Mother: "I will help you when you need help; you can start doing your homework in the room next to the kitchen."

Ben: "I'll need a lot of help doing some of the homework."

Mother: "I thought of a plan for doing homework. When you come home from school, you can do whatever you want until 4:00. At 4:00, come back to the kitchen with your homework assignment to do in the living room. This way, I can answer any questions you have. At 5:00, take a snack break and during this time I will review your homework. At 5:30 you will stop doing homework for the day as long as you do your best. Is this plan ok with you."

Ben: "Ok, I can live with that."

Mother: "That's great. We can always work together to get the job done. Shall we start today so you won't get further behind?"

Ben: "I don't want to start until after it's dark so I can play outside."

Mother: "I can go along with that this time."

The first step was for the mother to clearly identify the child's problem. "Homework is too hard and too much." Once the child recognize that his mother understand his concern, he is more willing to listen to suggestions. The mother responded first to the main concern "it is too hard": by suggesting that she could be available to answer questions and help during homework time by having him do the work in the room next to the kitchen. In response to the second concern, "it is too much," the mother helped to structure the afternoon and break homework time into smaller parts. Sudden changes to an ADHD child cause anxiety and lead to resistance; asking his opinion about when to start this new plan gives him a feeling of control. When your child presents a problem:

Always establish a habit of reflection and considering all the options rather than black and white impulsive thinking. You are coaching the child to go through the steps of reflective thinking. "Ready, Fire, Aim!" is the impulsive response of most ADHD children.

What can parents do to improve the memory of their child?

1. Help your child to be more organized. They need this as a foundation for improved memory. Make sure he has a specific place for all his belongings, a set place for homework, a schedule and a neat clean room.
2. Teach your child to look at the person's face who is talking to him. Make sure he is seated close to the front of the class.
3. Encourage your child to ask the teacher to repeat information he did not understand.
4. An ongoing exercise should be to relate new information to something he already knows. Help him make connections to build long term memory.

► **DEALING WITH MULTIPLE PROBLEMS:**

Children with ADHD exhibit many symptoms; some more serious than others. Those that can put the child in danger or negatively impact other family members must have the highest priority. To train and coach your child to develop his coping skills, you will want to improve his strengths and weaknesses. By understanding and discussing these issues with your spouse and your child's teachers, you will be in the best position to be an effective leader and have confidence in your decisions. Clearly, a child who wanders off or impulsively runs across the street needs to have those mental skills developed first.

Do not get discouraged when the list of your child's problems is quite long. Keep in mind that you can succeed but the problems will not go away overnight. However, many issues are related to each other and when one brain function improves, related symptoms are diminished. In other words, when there is an improvement in concentration, not one but many symptoms of poor concentration will diminish. Prioritizing the issues will keep you from being caught in struggles over relatively trivial matters. As a parent-coach you always want to think about how to capitalize on your child's strengths. Always praise your child for a job well done. This will build his confidence and self esteem.

▶ **LEARN TO PRIORITIZE PROBLEMS:**

Learning to prioritize problems, actions and goals in life are important for everyone and even more so for the ADHD child. Is cleaning the room more important than participating in organized sports? No. Both are important responsibilities –one to the family and one to his teammates. I'm sure you would have no problem prioritizing whether to return a phone call to your boss or your friend first. An ADHD child's needs usually must be addressed before preparing supper or any other responsibilities or you face disrupting the entire family.

▶ **BEGIN NEGOTIATING WITH YOUR CHILD:**

Many of the disagreements or disruptions with your ADHD child come when he is expected to do household chores, homework or adhere to household rules. Negotiation is a powerful tool in these activities of daily living and helps improve the deficiency in thinking and organizational skills in the ADHD child. The best way to approach negotiation is for both sides to gain something from the negotiations. A give and take discussion with your child should result in the feeling that you both gained something and your relationship is better. As your interactions with your child become more successful and productive, your communication will also improve and you will engender trust and respect from your child. Understand your child before you help him understand you. Being consistent, calm and keeping your promises will serve as a base for a positive relationship. The level of communication and trust increases if your child feels you really understand him. You must avoid insults, put downs and overreaction regardless of your child's behavior. Remember, you are his parent and the one he relies on as a source of comfort, motivation and trust.

Negative behavior your child exhibits reveals insecurity, anxiety or depression. It is a projection of his fears that he is unlovable and no one can protect him in times of stress. You have to listen to him and let him talk first. Do not interrupt. One way to show that you are listening and understanding is to repeat in your own words what he has told you. Try to summarize it. "I know you hate to do homework and it's hard, but in order to succeed, you must continue to learn. Let's try to find a way to make the homework easier."

▶ **YOUR MOST IMPORTANT GOAL AS A COACHING PARENT:**

Your love for your child is unconditional and does not depend on good or bad behavior; he needs to know that. He should feel certain that he can count on you 100% and the whole family is on the same team, and pulling for his success. Give lots of preemptive hugs and praise. Look for actions that can justify praise. Hug him and say: "You have been a wonderful big brother today and a big help to me." or "Wow, you did a great job cleaning your room." These simple acts will help strengthen his belief in himself and instill a feeling of confidence that is essential in helping him overcome many of the challenges he will face in life.

▶ **IMPORTANT POINTS TO REMEMBER:**

- To be an effective "coaching parent" you must always set clear limits and rules, be firm and decisive once your decision is made. Never waiver. Be consistent.
- The coaching staff, i.e. the mother and father and other caregivers must communicate the same expectations to the child and agree on the methods of discipline and rules. No conflicting messages.
- When giving directions, be succinct, simple and clear.

- Be proactive. Plan your actions with your child to reduce conflict.
- Clarify each goal and plan step by step what is needed to achieve the goal you have set. The journey to reach the goal is as important as the goal itself in developing a positive atmosphere in the family and a higher degree of confidence.
- Prioritize a list of problems or conflicts that you feel your child needs to resolve. Deal with the most pressing, painful or dangerous issues first.
- Negotiation is the most effective way to resolve conflict. Find a solution that does not overwhelm the child. For example, if a child has been given a particularly long homework assignment, break it into shorter segments. Guide him through difficult parts. Allow for breaks and let him ventilate his frustration.
- Empathize with his difficulties and offer less frustrating methods to help him complete his task.
- Avoid threats, anger, overreaction and impulsive actions or remarks regardless of your child's behavior.
- Your love and the family's full support will form a strong base to strengthen your child's emotional stability.
- Your child must feel unconditional love from his parents that is not contingent on his behavior.
- Look for behavior to praise.

Chapter 5

EFFECTIVE PARENTING

$\mathbf{A}$ child's perception of the world around him is essential in building his confidence and *character*. It isn't the parent's intentions that count, but rather a child's knowledge that he is loved unconditionally. If a child feels that love is withdrawn every time he misbehaves or disappoints his parents, his emotional sense of security is threatened. *Most emotional problems adults deal with stems from a perception of love withheld.* When children are criticized from an early age, their self-esteem and confidence erodes. Statistically, parents makes 5–9 times more negative comments to their children than positive ones, and the relationship between them is undermined as a result. Often parents criticize thoughtlessly or because they actually believe it is "constructive."

However, true constructive criticism leaves the person feeling better and more capable.

If criticism diminishes self-esteem and confidence, then it is detrimental.

"Rules of Engagement":

1. Protect your child's self-esteem and feelings of self-worth at all costs; begin any discussion of problems with a loving

statement. Combine any negative statement that must be made with a positive.

2. Do not dredge up the past; focus on what can be done now.

3. Replace "*You* make me so mad" with a statement about the problem. Begin the process of improvement in behavior/ school performance, etc.: "With such a great kid that we love so much, I can't understand these grades/behavior/ etc. I know this makes us both feel sad. Let's think together. We can always solve problems when we work together as a team."

4. A parent must also be a coach. When you offer to help, be prepared to come up with constructive advice, to show the child how to improve. Be specific about what has to change and how to accomplish the goals you have set.

5. Assume your child wants to succeed and do a good job. He does not disappoint you deliberately. The problem is immaturity, inadequate skills or some other influence that can be corrected.

6. Keep your cool. Be clear and constructive. Build your child up rather than erode his feelings of self worth. Rule #1: Always make a positive statement before a negative one. Fear of failure and rejection, acquired during childhood, has an enduring impact on the personality and attitudes of the adults they will become. Just remember, when you are thinking, "I have to teach this kid a lesson," make sure it's a positive one.

▶ **POSITIVE MEMORIES OF CHILDHOOD EXPERIENCES:**

Adult Case History: Effective Parenting during Childhood
Koby was born to a middle class family. His father, a small independent businessman, was busy most of the time running his company. He would leave early in the morning, often before the

children were up, and return so late at night that the time they spent together was very limited. Koby's mother, Ruth, worked as a secretary in a local law office and was responsible for most of the family matters. She was the one who met with the teachers, helped with school projects and homework and provided structure and guidance to the children. When he was four years old, during holidays and family get-togethers, Koby overheard his aunt saying: "Koby is just unstoppable. I don't know how you handle him. He never seems to sit still." His mother responded, "I wish I could have so much energy."

Koby recalled this memory 36 years later in my office. A highly successful businessman who recently sold his company, he came to my office to find out if he suffers from ADHD like his son, who was diagnosed a few weeks earlier.

"I was known as the kindergarten superman," he said. "I was very good in sports and always found a way to shine in this arena. I got a lot of positive re-enforcement from playing and excelling at sports."

(*Achievement in after-school activities boosts self-esteem*)

Koby's situation in school was entirely different.

"My first grade teacher called my mother for the first time the second week of the school year complaining that I couldn't sit quietly. Then came the complaints that I interrupt the class without being called on, don't follow the teacher's instructions, or instructions must be repeated several times. My teacher tried to help by developing a point system to reward good behavior. My next teacher complained that I was never organized and seldom finished a homework assignment. From then until my last year in elementary school, my mother became a regular at school meetings to try to explain my behavior and work on a solution to reduce the difficulties. But my grades were poor, and by the end of the 5th grade, the teacher suggested that I repeat the year. After much discussion, the principal accepted my mother's suggestion that I enter a remedial summer program to prepare for the 6th grade. While I had a miserable time in school, I was highly successful in after-school activities. By playing sports, I could forget all my problems. My feelings of being stupid and a failure disappeared when I was on the field."

(*A supportive home environment despite problems is essential.* Parents do not have to be perfect.)

"My home life was not easy for me during these years. Although my mother and father had a good relationship, there were arguments, mostly about my behavior. I felt different from my brother and sister. They had lots of friends and social activities, while although I excelled at sports, very few of my teammates were close friends.

Mornings were also difficult for me. When my brother and sister were almost ready to leave for school, I was just getting my schoolbag organized. My mother usually had to help me by making a list of things to do every morning. This list was posted in several places to help me organize myself. Homework was the worst, though. I had more fights and conflict with my mother about homework than everything else put together. Completing a homework assignment took me much more time than it took my sister even though she was younger than I. Any noise, phone call, TV program or conversations could easily ruin my concentration. My mother tried to create a quiet place for me to study. I don't recall any severe punishments, but several times I lost privileges and I clearly remember one evening when she said I would have to talk to my father about the homework. By the time my father arrived at home, I was very anxious. He gave me a warm hug as always and we went to his room for privacy He told me that he loved me very much and that he was very proud of me. Every weekend when he saw how hard I tried and how well I did on the soccer field, he would tell my grandparents and his friends how much fun it is to watch me play and how proud he was. But he said that we have a problem because my resistant to doing homework caused my mother stress. Because homework is a part of school and can not be changed, he asked me to work with my mother to find the best way to finish this task every day.

So I really tried. I don't remember any further talks with my father about homework until high school. I managed to limp along."

▶ **FOSTERING SELF-ESTEEM AND CONFIDENCE:**
"Frequent fights often involved struggles with my brother and sister over the TV. I enjoyed watching TV by myself because I had total control. Of course my brother and sister also wanted to watch TV, so we fought over control of the TV program. I remember one afternoon, my mother called me into the kitchen and said that she had a nice surprise for me and took me to my father's workroom. On my father's desk next to his computer was a new computer game.

She told me that I would have to share it with my brother and sister but for now, you can play with it. This was the beginning of a change in my life. At the time, very few families had computers at home. My sister had no interest in it and my older brother used it only when one of his friends came to visit. I was lucky that I was able to use the computer by myself without the regular fights. I started to play games and became quite good at them, to the point where I could beat everyone including my father. My father was impressed and suggested I go to a children's class in computers. I started to attend and really enjoyed it."

As our office visit was coming to an end, I told Koby that based on his childhood history, there was a good possibility that he had the same condition as his son since there is a strong genetic component to his condition, but more information was necessary. I expressed interest in hearing the rest of the story and gave him a questionnaire – the Adult ADHD Self Report Scale. Looking at his answers along with the childhood history helped determine the diagnosis.

► **WHAT DOES IT TAKE FOR ADHD CHILDREN TO SUCCEED IN LIFE?**

The history of Koby's childhood is a good example of how parents can help and guide their child from grammar school through high school, even with some behavior problems. It's unfortunate that Koby had to spend years of his childhood under-achieving and feeling stupid. Even though he graduated from high school with below average grades, he entered adult life with strengths and skills that helped him establish a stable family and build a successful business. Koby is one of several cases of adults with ADHD who were able to succeed quite remarkably in different arenas of life without medication or professional intervention. We know of many highly successful physicians, lawyers, artists, athletes, actors and others who exhibited symptoms of ADHD during their childhood and became very successful adults with ADHD. However, there are many more who do not reach their potential.

Examining the history of this group shows a pattern of action, responses and attitudes of parents toward these children. And it seems that parental attitude and action is what makes the difference.

► **WHAT PARENTS CAN DO TO LEAD THEIR ADHD CHILD TO SUCCESS:**

The following factors were present in Koby's case:

1. Koby's parents accepted his condition as a fact and they made the appropriate adjustments.
2. They showed consistent love and a positive attitude regardless of his behavior. Koby's strong memory as a child of a positive remark his mother made about his constant activity demonstrates his general perception of his parents' positive attitude. Even in kindergarten, his mother tried to create a positive image of Koby by labeling him "superman." The problem was presented in a positive light, but not ignored or denied. These are the interactions that Koby remembers

from his childhood. His father's first statement when dealing with his exasperating behavior was, "You know I love you and am really proud of you."

3. Only *after* a positive loving statement did Koby's father show disapproval of Koby's behavior and insist on improvement. There were very few times that Koby reported negative comments by his parents. Considering everything, their responses toward him were wise, quite positive and consistent.

4. Living in a stable family situation greatly contributes to the feelings of security and comfort for the ADHD child. He needs this security for his emotional growth. In this group of highly successful adults with ADHD, the positive influence of the parents was an extremely important factor..

5. The parents re-enforced their child's strengths and helped motivate him to overcome his weaknesses. These parents searched for activities where the ADHD child could excel and build his self-esteem to compensate for the tasks that were difficult for him. In Koby's case, his father strongly supported involvement in sports and sent him to computer classes where he knew he could excel. The result was outstanding and despite the difficulties Koby was having during high school, his computer skills and success in sports diluted the negative feedback he was getting from most of his high school teachers and some of his peers.

6. Almost all highly successful adults with ADHD report above average success in some activity outside of school during their high school years.

7. Many highly successful adults with ADHD report honing other skills outside of school. Many dancers, actors, radio and TV personalities with ADHD report spending hours in all kinds of after school activities that gave them positive re-enforcement in areas where they were able to excel and develop strong positive self esteem.

▸ HOW TO DEVELOP SELF-ESTEEM IN THE ADHD CHILD:

Praise for positive behavior is much more effective in influencing and molding your child than punishment for bad behavior. When you do have something negative to say, begin with a positive statement. "I know you want to do your best so we need to work together to find the best way to...."

Successful ADHD adults were able to develop a high level of self-esteem. Careful analysis of what helped them to develop this self-esteem reveals several contributing factors:

1. Warm relationship with an adult in addition to their parent. In most cases, this adult was a sport coach, teacher or leader in a youth group.

2. Connectedness was a common finding in childhood histories. As children, ADHD adults were connected with some group that allowed them to feel very proud of their abilities and accomplishments. The activity conducted with the group was usually after school hours, on weekends and during vacations. The positive feelings that stemmed from being a part of these groups compensated for the negative feelings they were encountering in school.

3. Development of special skills or talents was always a key to the success of these children. Parents were able to identify some interest or talent and capitalize on it.

4. Skill development through programs that developed their special interests, skills or talents were successful as all reported going through different stages or levels in enhancing their abilities. Completing one level or stage of training successfully and then moving up to the next stage contributed a sense of confidence and helped them develop some order in their thinking process. Another benefit was the planning skills that most started to acquire. These are skills missing in most ADHD children.

Understanding Koby's childhood history and analyzing

other successful adult ADHD childhood experiences set a good example for parents facing similar hurdles.

▶ **IMPORTANT POINTS TO REMEMBER:**

- Accept the condition your child has and learn to adapt to it.
- Show constant love and a positive attitude toward your child, regardless of his behavior or actions, and look for opportunities to praise him.
- Re-enforce your child's strengths to help him develop self-esteem.
- Having a stable warm relationship with parents, in addition to another significant relationship, helps the child to establish positive self-esteem.
- Being connected to some group activity on a consistent basis after school hours or on weekends helps a child develop self worth and a sense of belonging.
- Help your child develop special skills or talents to give him a strong sense of accomplishment.
- Attaining a high level of skill in activities that stimulate brain growth and development will not only build self-confidence and enhance planning skills but will overcome the neurotransmitter deficiency present in ADHD.
- Your child can be among the successful. It is possible to eliminate this disorder and thrive.
- You have the keys to help your child succeed.
- If you have difficulty expressing warmth and praise, the probability is high that at least one of your parents did too. You have choice: you can have the same relationship with your children... or not. Give him the gifts of high self-esteem and confidence; make sure your child knows he has unconditional love.
- If people remark that you are a negative cup-is-half-empty person, make it your top priority to change.

Chapter 6

TREATMENT METHODS FOR CHILDREN WITH ADHD

▶ **A CHRONIC CONDITION THAT CAN LAST A LIFETIME WITHOUT TREATMENT:**

If the symptoms of ADHD are not brought under control, it may be necessary for parents and/or children to seek psychotherapy for emotional distress such as depression or anxiety.

To treat a child with ADHD, at least five modalities of treatment can be used at different stages and with different combinations during a child's life.

▶ **IS MEDICAL TREATMENT EFFECTIVE?**

Yes. In most accurately diagnosed cases, the use of medication can be useful in the beginning. The drug class that includes methylphenidate (Ritalin) is the best known of this type of medication. It is effective in reducing the symptoms in about 70–80% of the cases. These are among the best studied and safest medications used in pediatrics. This does not mean medical monitoring is not required. When medication is reported not to "work", it is often because the dose was too small to be effective. The use of medication remains very controversial to parents. Despite the proven record in hundreds of studies, it is understandable that many parents are reluctant to use any medication on a daily basis in a young child.

The purpose of this book is to empower parents to take charge of their child's progress and to use natural brain stimulation to overcome ADHD. If the child is encouraged and motivated, the need for medication should be eliminated completely as the brain grows and develops. Furthermore, these changes can be permanent. With methylphenidate (Ritalin), the symptoms return as soon as the medication is stopped.

Will medication stop all the symptoms?

No. Despite improvement in concentration, focus, impulse control and academic work, medication will do nothing for social skills, frustration tolerance and taking responsibility. Nor can medication compensate for a home without clear rules and direction or poor thinking skills.

What happens when medication is stopped?

The same symptoms of inattention and hyperactivity will return. Medication does *not* make permanent changes in brain function. Only in the last few years has research revealed the very important connection between vigorous mental and physical exercises and stimulation of the brain to increase neuronal connections and synapses to support these activities. The more skillful the person becomes, the more effective the brain connections are. Medication is very useful in the beginning of treatment, but as lagging skills improve, medication can be decreased and finally eliminated.

▶ IS PSYCHOTHERAPY EFFECTIVE TREATMENT?

Psychotherapy by itself is less effective. However, because many children with ADHD also exhibit anxiety or depression, the use of psychotherapy to alleviate these accompanying symptoms is effective. Individual psychotherapy does not seem to contribute to improving ADHD symptoms. However, certain group therapy processes may help the ADHD child by giving him an opportunity to get feedback from other group members and improve his social skills.

▶ **IS BEHAVIORAL THERAPY EFFECTIVE TREATMENT?**

Yes, in some cases. Behavioral therapy is a method of correcting behavioral problems by using a reward system to encourage positive behavior and discourage inappropriate behavior. It has been used extensively to improve children's behavior, social relationships and general adjustment in school and at home. This method may sometimes be effective in dealing with the management of violation of house rules, failure to complete homework or household chores and other undesirable behavior. It is most successful in young children aged four to ten. This type of treatment has been the standard approach for children with ADHD. The reason many parents report that they fail to see any real change once this type of treatment is terminated is that ADHD is a cognitive (thinking) problem and *not* a behavioral one. The two biggest problems with behavioral therapy are how to get the desired behavior to continue when the reward is discontinued and how to get the desired behavior in new similar situations. Behavioral therapy has only limited use in the treatment of ADHD. The ultimate goal is to develop internal motivation. That will come from the good feelings following the acquisition of a new ability and empowerment from solving problems with one's own mental resources. This is the reason cognitive therapy is a powerful tool; it is addressing lagging thinking skills.

▶ **IS COGNITIVE THERAPY AN EFFECTIVE METHOD TO TREAT ADHD CHILDREN?**

Yes. Cognitive therapy can help a person resolve emotional, social or other conflicts by approaching the issue rationally to find the best solution. The goal of cognitive therapy is to have the child think through his problems, rather than acting impulsively on the first thing that comes to mind. The best cognitive therapies are Collaborative Problem Solving (CPS) developed by Dr. Ross W. Greene and Mediated Learning Experience (MLE) developed by Dr. Reuven Feuerstein.

Since ADHD *is a thinking disorder, only by improving thinking skills will the symptoms of* ADHD *be diminished.*

The following chapters will teach parents how they can use CPS effectively to help their ADHD child. This kind of therapy has been highly successful and led to resolution of ADHD symptoms. Much more about CPS in later chapters.

► WHY IS BRAIN EXERCISE THERAPY (BET) EFFECTIVE FOR ADHD?

Brain Exercise Therapy is a method of increasing the number and complexity of brain neuronal connections. The use of BET is so new in the treatment of ADHD that we do not have all the answers. However, we do know it is a powerful tool for neuronal growth and improving thinking skills. I can report to you from personal experience, as well as from many of my patients, the tremendous benefits of BET.

With BET, there is a dramatic increase in the complexity of brain function in the specific areas where the ADHD child is deficient and results are real changes in both the actual weight and sophistication of the brain. This is a major breakthrough in the successful treatment of ADHD symptoms.

These exercises have been shown to physically enhance the interconnectedness of brain neurons, specifically in the areas where the brain is underdeveloped or deficient in neurotransmitters. It is very effective when used in combination with cognitive therapy and medication in the early stages. (The goal is to gradually decrease medication as the brain grows and matures).

▶ **HOW TO TEACH YOUR CHILD TO MANAGE TRANSITION EFFECTIVELY:**

Transition is very difficult for children with ADHD. Switching from a fun activity to one they consider boring often causes major conflict. Switching from playing to homework or house chores, or from TV time to dinnertime or bedtime, will often cause conflict. To minimize the child's reaction to such changes, you can prepare the child for transition.

1. Give your child advance notice of the change in activity that will soon take place. "We are going to leave the park in five minutes. Take your last few turns on the slide."
2. Ask your child to repeat what you just said.
3. When the time arrives for the transition, say "I told you several minutes ago that we will leave the park in a few minutes. We are leaving now. Let's go."
4. Praise your child for following through. If the child continues to resist, repeat step 2. Immediately follow up with step 3. "We are leaving. Let's go."

Examples of managing transition time:

Mother: "Ben, you have been watching TV for 45 minutes. In 15 minutes, we are leaving Grandmother's house to return home."

Ben: "No, I don't want to! Why now?"

Mother: "Ben, repeat what I just said."

Ben: "You said we have to leave".

Mother: "Ben, I want you to listen now carefully so you can repeat after me. We are leaving to go home. In 15 minutes we are going home."

Ben: "You said in 15 minutes we are going home".

Mother: "Ok, I am coming back to remind you when you have five more minutes. Then I want you to turn off the TV without any debate and tell your grandmother goodbye."

Ben: "Ok."

Mother: (10 minutes later) "Ben, in five minutes it is time to go home. Please turn off the T V and tell your grandmother goodbye."

Ben: "I wish I could watch T V longer."

Mother: "No, we are leaving now."

Ben: (Turns off the T V and speaks to his grandmother).

Another example of managing transition:

Michael and a friend are playing in his room.:

Mother: "Michael, in 30 minutes, supper will be ready and Sam will have to go home."

Michael: "I don't want to eat."

Mother: "I will come back in 20 minutes to remind you that in 10 minutes Sam will have to go home. We expect you to be at the table."

Michael: "We are in the middle of a game!"

Mother: "You can put the game aside and continue it tomorrow. Did you hear what I said?"

Michael: "Yes."

Mother: "What did I say?"

Michael: "You will remind me in 20 minutes and we can finish the game tomorrow."

Mother: "Great. So you have 30 minutes to play."

Mother: (In 20 minutes) "In 10 minutes Sam will have to go home and you must come to the table."

Michael: "No way. We are in the middle of the game."

Mother: "You have 10 minutes and that's all."

Mother: (10 minutes later) "Time's up. Sam has to go home. You can finish the game tomorrow. "

Michael: "Just ten more minutes, pleeeze."

Mother: "No Michael. That's it. Come to the table now. Sam has to go home."

Michael: (Somewhat unhappily) "All right. Sam, let's finish tomorrow. Come home with me after school."

A defined schedule, organizational skills, clear rules and consistency are the bread and butter of the treatment program. They serve as the first step in the process of overcoming ADHD.

(A full list of cognitive skills to be developed, will be discussed in detail).

▸ **IMPORTANT POINTS TO REMEMBER:**

The reason the implementation of all the different treatment modalities simultaneously is so important: The cortex is arranged in three layers; we want to stimulate growth and development from the top, down and from the bottom, up.

- Five modalities of treatment can be used in different situations in the child's life. Medication, psychotherapy, behavior therapy, cognitive therapies and brain exercise therapy.
- Organization and consistency are crucial.
- The use of medication such as methylphenidate is effective in more than 70% of cases by reducing the severity of symptoms and improving the quality of the child's life. However, there are many symptoms such as immaturity and deficient social skills that are not influenced by medication.
- Ritalin and other similar medication make no permanent changes in brain function; as soon as the drug is stopped, the symptoms return.
- Psychotherapy is used mostly in cases of depression, anxiety or other associated conditions of the child with ADHD.
- Behavioral therapy is useful in improving a child's social relationships and his general adjustment in school and in the home. Best results are achieved when it is used with children ages 4–10.
- Coaching your child in the development of social skills is very effective.
- Cognitive therapy is highly effective in enriching thinking skills.
- Brain exercise therapy dramatically increases the number

and complexity of neuronal connections in the part of the brain where ADHD children are deficient. It must be done at least five days a week, but if you make it fun, that will not be an issue.

Chapter 7

COGNITIVE THERAPY

▶ **UNDERSTANDING ADHD THINKING:**

The development of the behavior therapy program to manage misbehavior of children with ADHD was based partially on the assumption that ADHD behavior was a result of inconsistent discipline. It was thought that inconsistent discipline, low supervision, or inflexible rigid discipline, all contributed to a child's misbehavior. Therefore, the goal of behavior therapy was to teach adults to be more consistent, more involved, much more positive, and less rigid in order to help their child change behave more productively and desirably. Follow up of parents who received training to implement this kind of program showed that a substantial number of parents did not fully comply with the implementation of behavioral therapy or simply dropped out of treatment.

Taking aim at the 50% of children who do not benefit, Dr. Ross W. Greene recommended the use of alternative strategies to help parents deal more effectively with ADHD children. ("The Explosive Child" by Ross W. Greene, PhD. 1998). This alternative strategy developed into a new model of cognitive therapy: The Collaborative Problem Solving Approach (CPS). New brain research has helped us understand not only the causes of ADHD, but also its actual impact within the brain and the consequences.

This mild biological malfunction of the young brain causes the child to lack specific skills that would help him cope effectively with frustration, problem solving and flexibility. We now understand that the emotional difficulties of the ADHD child, such as lacking the ability to cope with stress and frustration, is due to cognitive limitations and *not* behavior.

Unless treatment is implemented to correct these biological deficits, the child simply cannot control his behavior. It is not because he's spoiled or because the parents are too lenient. Expecting a child to modify behavior without treatment intervention is just like blaming a diabetic for not producing enough insulin. This is why motivational strategies and behavior modification are *not* very effective when used alone.

This insight was a major breakthrough in the treatment of ADHD. Now that we fully understand that specific cognitive skills in an ADHD child are not fully developed, we can understand why motivational strategies were not as effective as expected. They simply did not address the biological deficiencies. Learning disabilities, like reading, do not respond effectively to reward and punishment for the same reason; the cause is biological. The child's delayed development of skills necessary to solve problems and show patience is a learning disorder of a specific type and causes the child's misbehavior.

When cognitive demands are placed on the child that outstrip the child's capacity to respond, you can be sure misbehavior will be the result. After correcting the biological deficit with medication, a child can learn the skills that will enable him to solve problems and not to impulsively choose the first option that comes to mind. He will be able to deal with sudden shifts in activities and tolerate frustration. With the natural changes that result from the daily use of CPS, BET and other effective means of therapeutic intervention, the amount of dopamine in the brain can be brought to normal levels and, at that point, methylphenidate is no longer needed.

The area of the brain that is responsible for management and control of our thinking and emotion is not fully developed in the ADHD child. Often by the end of adolescence, this area normalizes, but in a significant number of cases, medication must continue throughout life unless BET and cognitive CPS are used intensively. *Keep in mind that, without intervention, your child will go through many of his formative years with unnecessary anxiety, never reaching his academic potential and with relentless underperformance and criticism even if he does eventually outgrow his ADHD deficiencies. Do not for one minute think this will not leave an emotional scar.*

The part of the brain that houses these deficiencies is responsible for many of our cognitive functions. We see the impact of these deficiencies in five areas of cognitive function. The lagging skills in each of these areas prevent a child from responding to challenges productively and push him toward explosive behavior.

► **WHAT ARE THE FIVE THINKING DOMAINS THAT ARE NOT FULLY DEVELOPED?**

Executive Skills:

Several cognitive skills have been associated with this neurological pathway. Working memory allows us to store events in our minds to be used later on to help make the proper decisions and problem solve. Decision making and planning are below age level.

Organization and planning skills:

Organizational skills in ADHD children are deficient, but they can be "coached" and trained to develop these skills, which are critical in inhibiting impulses, generating solutions to problems and helping define the problems. The lack of a well-developed organizational system in the brain explains why the ADHD child is disorganized, absent-minded and impulsive. It also means the child is often unable to identify what frustrates him or think of more than one solution to a problem.

Inflexible thinking:

Changes in plans and new requests are often rejected by ADHD children. Thinking clearly will allow a child to separate his emotional state of anger or frustration from facts. When he can access all the information from his memory bank, more potential solutions are available to him. The impulsive child picks the first solution that comes to his mind, which frequently is not the best. Thinking clearly and calmly can be achieved with the proper training of thinking skills.

Shifting one's cognitive set, i.e. changing from one activity to another requires flexibility. For example, a child who is playing in the yard will respond slowly to a request to come inside. When finally entering the house, he may continue to act as if he were still outside running wildly or climbing on the furniture.

Rules for behavior inside the house and outside are different, and this is a difficult transition for an ADHD child. As a parent you must keep this fact in mind as requests for change will cause stress and potential problems for a child.

A child can learn to handle transitions in activities in a productive way and adapt to new circumstances. By slightly modifying instructions, you can dramatically alter the level of conflict.

Language processing skills:

Lagging language processing skills can cause a child to have difficulty learning to deal with problems relating flexibility and frustration. Language is used to express thinking and communicate effectively. There are three specific areas where the language skills of an ADHD child are lagging.

Expression of emotion:

Many defiant, angry children do not have the basic vocabulary to express their feelings. These children will frequently say, "I hate you," "Go away," or "Leave me alone." "Bad Mommy." A hostile child elicits a predictable response in adults, which causes the child to become even more frustrated. The cycle is difficult to stop. The inability to recognize their own emotions causes a child to express all of them with the same reaction – an outburst of anger.

Expression of their needs:
A child must be able to express his needs in order to reduce stress and prevent impulsive behavior. When a child's needs and wants are expressed clearly, the level of frustration and anger decreases. Without these skills, a child quickly becomes irritable, angry and explosive.

Solving problems:
Children with poor language skills will have difficulty accessing past solutions to learn from them because past experiences and memories are stored in language form. By teaching children a basic emotional vocabulary, they will be better equipped to express their needs and access past solutions stored in their brain.

Improvement of language skills will also help a child understand what was said to him and allow him to respond to questions without excessive delay.

Emotion Regulation Skills:
When a child is irritable, agitated or cranky, he tends to become more easily frustrated. He may carry this emotion from one event to another unrelated event. The result is an anxious child, who may cry, throw tantrums or shout. These emotional reactions are triggered by a problem or challenge they cannot not immediately solve. You will be aware that the emotional outburst is completely out of proportion to the cause, i.e. crying for long periods of time over a minor insult or frustration.

A lack of emotional regulation skills reduces the capacity for clear thinking, which in turn prevents effective problem solving. Disproportionate anxiety is another symptom of ADHD and makes clear rational thought more difficult just when clear thinking is most necessary.

▶ WHAT COGNITIVE AND FLEXIBILITY SKILLS ARE MISSING?

Many children find it easier to function by using rigid and inflexible thinking because everything is black and white. The delays in development of flexible thinking skills may be an attempt to reduce general anxiety by thinking in very concrete terms.

Often these kids get "stuck" in a belief system and it can be a blow to self-esteem when these set ways of thinking are challenged. Volumes have been written about how to re-structure inflexible belief systems. The parent should always gently question a misguided belief system.

For example:

Child: "I can't do this puzzle (my homework/read as well as…). I'm stupid."

Parent: "You think you're stupid because you can't do this puzzle?"

Child: "Yes. And the kids in school laughed at me because I lost my place when I was reading."

Parent: "Well, I think you're pretty smart. Look how quickly you can do math problems. Your teacher said you were one of her best math students. How can you be stupid if you are so good at math? And just think what a great soccer player you are! Maybe you are just too impatient to think about the puzzle. Why don't you leave it until after supper and then we'll do the puzzle together.

…or

Another example of "black and white" thinking:

Child: My teacher hates me!

Parent: "You think your teacher hates you?"

Child: "She does hate me. She really does."

Parent: "Just last week you were telling me how nice she is."

Child: "Well, now she hates me. And she's so mean."

Parent: "What happened in class today?"

Child: "I don't want to talk about it. And I'm never going back to school."

Parent: "Let's think about this together. Maybe your teacher had a reason to be upset."

Child: "All I did was throw a pencil to Ben."

Parent: "You threw a pencil to Ben."

Child: "Yes."

Parent: "Most teachers would be upset. Let's think together of how to solve this problem. Can you think of a solution?"

Child: "No."

Parent: "Maybe tomorrow you could go to her class early in the morning and apologize."

Child: "No. I can't. I won't."

Parent: "Well, maybe there's another way to apologize."

Child: "How?"

Parent: "You used to write notes to your big sister when she was upset with you."

Child: (Thinking). "Well… I am pretty good at writing. I could try that and just put it on her desk and leave before she gets there."

Parents: "That's a great idea!" See how we always find a solution when we think things through together."

What are the social skills that are missing?

Many ADHD children are emotionally immature for their age and therefore find social interaction with their peers difficult. Some are lacking the skills required to start a conversation with others, or enter a group activity or share. They do not realize the impact of their actions on others and often misinterpret the reaction and responses of others toward them. Understanding parents can help their children master this and other undeveloped social skills. You can be a valuable emotional mirror for your child and reflect back to them how they come across to others in a meaningful way. You can also use other children's behavior to make a point: "Look how Jake refuses to share the ball with Ben. That's why Ben doesn't want to play with him anymore. Everyone wants friends who are generous and willing to share."

Parent's reaction to lagging cognitive skills:

Parents are a major factor in influencing the character and personality of their children. They can have a tremendous impact on the degree of cognitive skills their ADHD child will develop. Socially competent children tend to have authoritative parents. These parents place limits, rules and controls on a child while providing warmth and nurturance. On the other hand, aggressive children tend to have permissive parents who respond to the children in an inconsistent manner and fail to set clear limits that are enforced all the time. Anxious children have dictatorial parents who set limits, rules and controls, but without warmth, praise or nurturing.

Coaching parents need to be in tune with their own strengths and weaknesses and be willing to modify their interactions with their child. Try to assess how often you praise your child compared to how often you find fault. You can train yourself to accentuate the positive and be physically and verbally affectionate, even if it's not your natural response. Coaching parents need to be acutely aware of how important their response to their ADHD child's deficiencies really is. *ADHD children need praise, warmth, understanding, patience and empathy.* Clearly the best coach for helping the ADHD child develop the skills he needs is the adult who spends the most time with him in the early years. That is why the mother is usually the person who will contribute the most to helping him overcome his weaknesses and improve his skills. If your child spends a significant part of his day with another adult, make sure they understand the problem and how they can be the most effective.

► **WHAT SHOULD PARENTS DO TO PREPARE FOR THEIR COACHING "CAREER"?**

Parents who are anxious about how their child is being perceived by others will react much more harshly to the child's misbehavior than parents who are aware of the causes of the child's problem, accept it and cease to view it as a reflection of parental incompetence. This is a source of major conflict in many homes with an ADHD child, where one parent blames the other for poor parenting. An irritable child who lives with impatient, inflexible parents will have a lot of additional stress compared to the same child who lives with parents who understand his limitations and work as a team to train him. Since ADHD is a condition that is 80% inherited, parents should do a personal assessment of their own symptoms of ADHD. Clearly a parent who struggles with executive function, emotional regulation and inflexible thinking is poorly prepared to deal with a child with the same weaknesses.

From the list below, you can arrange in order of importance the skills that your child needs to improve most. Every child is different and you are the one who knows which areas are making life miserable for your child and for you.

► **SKILLS THAT NEED TO BE DEVELOPED:**

Executive Skills:
- Handling transition
- Staying on topic
- Doing functions in order
- Sorting through thoughts
- Thinking through consequences of actions
- Considering a range of solutions
- Shifting from one mind set to another

Language Processing Skills:
- Verbally expressing emotions –frustration, sadness, happiness, etc.

- Expression of needs and concerns
- Clear expression of thoughts

Emotional Regulation Skills:
- Managing anxiety, depression, etc.
- Managing moods
- Limiting the emotional reaction to the cause
- Remaining positive in other areas of life when facing difficulties

Cognitive Flexibility Skills:
- Thinking in shades of color rather than black and white
- Adapts to changes appropriately
- Able to hear another point of view objectively
- Able to accept mistakes as a part of life

Social Skills:
- "Reads" verbal and nonverbal social cues
- Adapts well to group activities
- Understands how one's behavior affects others
- Seeks attention in productive positive way

► **FACTORS LEADING TO MISBEHAVIOR:**

Children face an increasing number of demands, challenges and expectations as they grow older. Social situations become more complex, teachers expect more mature behavior and life's challenges will often find the ADHD child falling further behind. It is so important that it is understood by parents and teachers. When demands placed upon an ADHD child exceeds his capacity to respond, you can be sure his reaction will be negative. This is a fact that must be understood by parents and teachers. To repeat, the ADHD child reacts in an inappropriate or unhelpful way because he lacks the cognitive skills to deal effectively with the demands placed upon him. It isn't because he's spoiled, selfish, etc. He simply does not have the skills. It is certainly not due to a lack of motivation. He may come across as manipulative and attention seeking, but it should be seen as a response to challenges he cannot meet.

Recognizing the five areas or pathways where the child is experiencing poorly developed skills below his age level will help us identify potential problems. Since each child demonstrates different degrees and types of difficulties, each child must be assessed individually. Some ADHD children are very charming and extroverted, and social skills are less of a problem for them than risk taking, acting out, disorganization, impulsive behavior, etc. Often parents can identify the source of past conflicts and trace the cause. Perhaps you will see that they all had some characteristic in common and usually it's something the child faces regularly such as homework, bedtime, reading, chores, relationships or siblings. The parents' goal should be to help the child develop thinking skills that will allow him to face the same or similar obstacles with improved results in the future.

▶ **CAN IMPROVING PROBLEM SOLVING SKILLS INCREASE BRAIN SIZE?**

Yes. Once it becomes clear that a child with ADHD has a deficit in cognitive skills, successful treatment can be implemented. Dr. Ross Greene, who developed a very effective approach to cognitive deficiencies, reported significant improvement using cognitive coaching in a number of studies. The parents and teachers who reported improvement also reported a reduction in parenting stress, improvement in parent-child interactions, and improved autonomy in the child.

The idea that coaching, training and practice improves thinking skills is confirmed by the work of Dr. Alvaro Pascual-Leone, a neuroscientist at Harvard Medical School. He showed that mental training had the power to increase the size of certain areas in the brain and increase neuronal connections. At this stage there have been no completed studies to show that this is the case in the brains of ADHD children. No doubt research will be done in the future, but one can extrapolate these studies to assume they apply to the ADHD child as well. Think of games to teach your child that involve thinking ahead, strategizing and memory, such as chess. If your child becomes proficient at chess and other activities that involve planning and thinking skills, you will see a general improvement in his thinking.

► **WHAT OPTIONS DO PARENTS HAVE TO SOLVE PROBLEMS?**

- Impose adult will. Often it is the father who acts decisively, feeling that it's his responsibility to solving the problem at hand. This approach can lead to results. However, the long-term benefit of this approach is questionable because similar problem tend to arise in the future. This method does not teach the child problem solving skills.
- The "Drop it" approach. To reduce tension and not upset the child further, the mother, in many cases, brings a soft approach to stop conflict. This approach reduces stress on both mother and child. However, no new skill is nurtured to help the child solve similar difficulties in the future.
- Collaborative problem-solving allows the parent and child to work through a solution together and develop flexibility and frustration tolerance.
- Use Brain Exercises (BET) to improve cognitive functions in all areas. Help you child develop expertise in targeted physical and mental exercises that address the cognitive weaknesses by the steps outlined in this book.
- A comprehensive approach will be the most effective. Parents can move gradually from an authoritarian approach to incorporate CPS, BET and other methods discussed here of stimulating the development of more sophisticated thinking skills.

▶ **IMPORTANT POINTS TO REMEMBER:**

- The child's delayed development of certain skills cause ADHD symptoms.
- Delayed skill development is a result of lagging thinking skills that can be overcome.
- To significantly enhance the capability to adequately respond to frustration and be flexible, skills in five domains need to be developed.

The domains are:
- Executive skills
- Language skills
- Social skills
- Emotional tolerance skills
- Cognitive skills
- An effective way to deal with inadequate problem solving skills and defiant oppositional behavior is by using Collaborative Problem Solving.
- BET enhances memory, planning, organization and thinking skills.
- A comprehensive approach will result in the development of more sophisticated mental functioning and medication can be gradually reduced and finally eliminated.
- Deficiency will vary with each child.

Chapter 8

COLLABORATIVE PROBLEM-SOLVING (CPS)

► **BIOLOGICAL BASIS FOR THE COLLABORATIVE PROBLEM SOLVING APPROACH:**

The medical consensus for decades has been that the brain is programmed; you are born with a finite (albeit huge) number of neurons and they do not grow or change significantly. Over the span of a lifetime, this number diminishes with age. In other words, hard wiring is present at birth. The brain has a huge number of unused neurons and with injury or disease, often these neurons could be activated to help in the repair process. Few considered the possibility that areas of the brain could change their basic functions completely, as for example, from vision to touch. The above theory was considered sacrosanct until now.

The brain is much more flexible than previously thought. With practice and training, the area of the brain that is stimulated actually grows! The physical size of this area of the brain increases as new neuronal connections are made. If you practice sudoku intensively, for example, a specific area of the brain used to solve these types of puzzles lights up and becomes physically larger.

In a like manner, if you encourage and develop a certain type of behavior, practice and repetition will yield similar results.

If you take this new knowledge and apply it to ADHD, the results are astounding. *Stimulation through learning and practicing in the areas of functioning where ADHD thought processes are weak will result in growth and development precisely in the areas where these skills are lagging.* This is a major breakthrough in neurology and has been clearly demonstrated at major medical centers in the United States and Europe. CPS and BET gradually reduce the need for medication as new neural pathways are generated. Other strategies will enhance this process.

▶ WHEN IS OPTIMAL TIME TO IMPLEMENT CPS?

The best time to begin coaching your child to develop his cognitive skills is when neither of you are experiencing undue levels of stress. If you were coaching a team, you would certainly not try new maneuvers during the game before practicing them in advance. In almost any endeavor in life, repetitive practice is essential to the learning process whether it's playing a musical instrument, sports or any other life skill.

▶ WHAT ARE THE FOUR STEPS NECESSARY TO IMPLEMENT CPS?

Empathy and Reassurance
Define the problem
Look at the options and consequences together
Help you child find the best solution and implement it

▶ HOW TO SHOW EMPATHY AND REASSURANCE:

Empathy and reassurance go a long way by acknowledging the child's feelings. An effective way to express empathy is by listening reflectively. You repeat or restate the child's comments. He will know you understand him or you can tell him what you observe that actually describes his feeling or state of mind.

For example:

Child (crying loudly): "I will never play with my sister again!"

Parent: "You seem very upset. Your sister upsets you."

In another instance the child returns home from playing with a friend very emotional and anxious:

Parent: "You seem very upset."

Child cries responding: "I do not want to talk about it."

Parent: "Something very upsetting happened while you were playing outside."

Child: "I got into a fight with one of my friends when we were playing soccer."

To help the child stay rational and begin to talk to you, effort must be directed toward creating an atmosphere of calm so that the second step of CPS can be initiated.

▶ HOW TO HELP THE CHILD DEFINE THE PROBLEM:

Defining the problem is the first step of the CPS approach. *The goal is to teach the child to say clearly exactly what is bothering him.* Sometimes the child does not understand why he is upset or why he misbehaves. Often he simply jumps to the first solution that comes to mind, i.e. "I never want to play with Sam again." Having the child express his real concerns is an important objective. With clear understanding of the problem the child is facing, the process of thinking and language skill development begins. After the child's concerns are identified and clearly expressed, only then can a parent state his concerns and point out the consequences of his "solution."

▶ HOW TO TEACH YOUR CHILD TO VERBALIZE HIS CONCERNS

To express his concern, the child needs to articulate it in words. For some children this first step of articulating his concerns into words is difficult.

For example:

Parent: "What's wrong?"

Child: "I don't know."

Parent: "You don't know or you don't know how to say it?"

Child: "Someone's always mad at me."

Parent: "Someone is always mad at you?"

This exchange is very common during the first few attempts.

Sometimes the child will not state a concern of specific difficulty, but will state the solution to his concern. "I'm not going to school." You may ask, "Why not?"

Scenario:

Child: "I don't want to do my homework".

Parent: "You do not want to do your homework. Why not"?

(The goal is to get a flow of conversation to identify the source of conflict that represents the child's concern).

Child: It's too hard.

Parent: "What is too hard for you?"

Since most ADHD child have specific cognitive skill deficiencies, each time they face the same challenge or demand they will respond in the same way. Parents should have a list of concerns or problems that have caused difficulties in the past. By using an educated guess and starting to name some of the more frequent trigger points as possible causes, one can help their child identify what causes his actions.

Parents: "Is it the loud music?"

Child: "No"

Parent: "Is it going out in the car"

Child: "No."

Parent: "Is it your brother?"

Child: "Yes."

This list of triggers should be posted in the house and carried by parents during the first stage of CPS so that the child will be able to identify concerns. Read the list to your child once he is calm. At the moment that he recognizes one of the triggers as a cause for his behavior, you have the beginnings of a successful plan. Some of the children will not be able to articulate their concerns because of poor language skills.

Parent: "Mary, what's going on? You haven't finished your homework."

Mary. "I don't know."

Mother: "Let's go over the list."

Mary: Ok, but it is not on the list.

Mother: "Is it my work in the kitchen?"

Mary: "Yes the kitchen."

Mother: "The kitchen seems to be the problem".

Mary: "Yes, the smell from the kitchen."

Mother: "The smell that comes from the kitchen bothers you"

Mary: "Yes."

By the time Mary and her mother were trying to resolve the new crisis, they were very familiar with the list of common triggers. However, in this particular case, since it was not a common one, it was not on the list.

▶ **HOW TO HELP YOUR CHILD TO UNDERSTAND AND VERBALIZE HIS CONCERNS:**

Teaching a child to express his concerns, even when the specific words elude him, can be productive. Teach him a few general phrases and coach him to apply them whenever he feels stressed. If he is unable to express his concern verbally, arm him with phrases, such as: "I need help." "Give me more time." "Something is bothering me." "I can't talk about it right now."

For example:

Mother: "Ben, how was soccer practice?"

Ben: "I don't know."

Mother: 'Sounds like something is bothering you."

99

Ben: "Yes, something is bothering me."

Mother: "Let's talk about it tonight after supper. We can always find a solution when we really think about it."

Having the child identify and articulate his concerns is only half of step one.

The other half is to let the parents express their concerns. In the beginning some parents announce their concerns by stating their solution to the problem, perhaps out of the belief that their concerns are more important than the child's. Often stating the solution to a concern indicates to the child that the parent does not really understand what his concerns are or his input is irrelevant.

▶ HOW TO LOOK FOR SOLUTIONS FOR THE PROBLEM:

Once both concerns are out in the open, the parent can invite the child to collaboratively brainstorm ideas that will contribute to a solution. All kinds of solutions should be suggested and evaluated. No solution at this stage should be rejected. This stage of the process allows the child to develop thinking skills. He should be involved in evaluating the problem and looking for a solution. The interaction between the child and the parent should leave no doubt that they are looking for a solution *together*. The way to emphasize this is by using such phrases as: "Let's work on this together." "How can we solve this problem?" "Let's think together how we can make things better."

The child should be the one to initiate a possible solution. A parent should say, "Tell me some of your suggestions," or "Do you know of some ways that might solve the problem?" Only after the child responds with several possible solutions should you say: "I have some ideas too. Would you like to hear them?"

In the beginning some of the children may have difficulty with thinking of solutions. In this case, do *not* impose a solution. You can ask, "What do you think of this idea for a solution?" or "How about X as a solution?"

▶ **HOW TO USE GENERAL COOPERATIVE SOLUTION AS A METHOD:**

You can explain to your child the benefits of finding a cooperative solution that is agreeable to both parent and child.

1. The parent and child should compromise to meet half way.
2. Teach your child to ask for help in dealing with certain problems.
3. Try to find a different way of solving a conflict or problem. The child must *actively participate* in the process of looking for solutions for the intervention to be successful.

How to choose the best solution for the problem:

The final step in collaborative problem solving is choosing the best available option. All solutions should be considered. There are only two factors that will determine the best choice. The solution should address and answer concerns of both sides. Neither side gets everything they ask but the solution must be acceptable and mutually satisfactory for both sides. The solution has to be realistic and feasible. In the eyes of the child there should be no such thing as a bad solution or idea. Good responses to a rejected solution by the parents could be: "This solution can work but it will be too difficult to accomplish it/take too long/etc. or "This solution does not answer both my concerns and your concerns." "This solution would solve the problem but you will lose your friendship."

The process of selecting a solution by reflecting on the feasibility and likely outcome of each possible solution will be training in thinking through an outcome and planning. As a good coach you may elaborate some specific solutions, for example, and state: "If you use this solution, 'A' could be the result; but if we opt for the other solution, 'B' will happen, so which one is best for you?"

After analyzing each potential solution, the best one can be chosen. Once a solution is chosen, the actual implementation of the solution should be carefully monitored. During the following few weeks, no new issues need to be introduced. All efforts should be focused on that problem and the way the child is implementing changes. Once some real changes are noticed, a different problem can be handled using the same method. There is a possibility that the child will not follow the plan and old behavior patterns will emerge. In this case, the parent needs to reintroduce the issue using the same practice approach. Now the focus needs to be on the last step of the method. Check to see that the solution chosen earlier is realistic and not too hard to carry out.

▶ **HOW TO USE A PROACTIVE APPROACH TO IMPLEMENT CPS:**

The most effective way to achieve a durable solution to the ADHD child's problems is by using a proactive plan to implement CPS. Parents need to identify the most common and troubling conflicts that cause the child's misbehavior. At the optimal time, when the child is not moody and not under stress or demands, a parent can say: "I have noticed that the problem we worked on together to find a solution still causes you some difficulties. What is going on?" or "I notice that every time, just before you start your homework, you are always upset." What's bothering you?"

You may wish to deal with new problems stating: "I've noticed that when you return from school on Mondays, you seem to be sad. What's up?" When the result of this approach to specific problems is not satisfactory, you need to get your child to review the solution that you decided to implement together .It's ok to make mistakes. Perhaps it was too difficult for the child to implement. You need to review all possible solutions again and select a solution that can be implemented in stages. With thinking disorders, the cognitive deficiencies of ADHD children will be improved step by step.

► HOW TO USE CPS APPROACH TO TRAIN FOR EXECUTIVE SKILL DEFICIENCIES?

This method can help parents train their ADHD child to improve many of his deficient cognitive skills and help develop better executive, language and social skills. Better organization and non-impulsive thinking can be accomplished by using the CPS approach. Defining a problem, reviewing past solutions as a model to solve present problems and evaluating the outcome of potential solutions, will all help improve some of the executive skills that are missing or not fully developed.

This pattern of thinking, i.e. defining a problem, reviewing possible solutions and evaluating the outcome of each, needs to be repeated until it is the natural first response. A major problem the ADHD child faces is dealing a shifting cognitive set. The sudden change from one set of rules to a new set is very problematic. An example of the need to shift from one set of cognitive behavior to another would be continuing playground once inside the house, moving from class to class, or moving from watching TV to the dinner table.

For example:

Parent: "It seems difficult for you to calm down when you come inside after playing outside. Can you think of a way to make it easier for you"?

Since the ADHD child has limited capacity to anticipate change, they fail to prepare in advance for the change. Using CPS will allow the child and his parents to anticipate regular shifts and prepare for it in advance.

Child: "I want to play outside."

Parent: "I know you like to play outside."

Child: "Yes, I can run as much as I want and nobody complains."

Parent: "Outside, no one complains about your running all the time."

Child: "You tell me to stop running as soon as I come home and making so much noise and then you always want me to do my homework. I hate doing homework."

Parent: "You are telling me that you feel free outside and you do not need to face doing your homework when you're playing."

Child: "I hate doing homework."

Parent: "You like to play outside and do not like doing your homework. (Help identify your child's problem by stating it in a clear way. Now it is your turn to state your concern or wishes.) "You cannot play outside all afternoon. Homework is a responsibility you have to complete for school." (Pause) "Did I understand your concern correctly?"

Child: Yes, I like to play outside and hate to do homework.

Parent: "Did you hear my concern?"

Child: "Yes."

Parent: "Can you repeat it?"

Child: "You said that I can not play all the afternoon outside since I have to do my homework."

Parent: "Let's think of ways to try to solve this problem together. Can you think of ways to make it easier for you?"

Child: "I can stay longer outside to play and when I come inside, I can watch TV until supper time."

Parent: "You get to play after you return from school for an hour. I'll let you stay an extra 30 minutes. When you come inside, you can go to your room for 10 minutes and then you have to do your homework. When you finish your homework, you can watch TV until supper time."

Child: "But sometimes school work is really hard and I need some help."

Parent: "You can do the work next to me in the kitchen so I can help you if needed. And afterwards you will have time to watch your favorite program."

Child: "Ok."

Parent: "Can you review what we both agreed as a solution?"

Child: "I get to play after school for one hour. When I come inside I can be

15 minutes in my room. Then I will start my homework next to you in the kitchen so you can help me when I need help. Then I can watch T V."

Parent: "I'm glad we found a solution. I will make a point to tell you 15 minutes before you have to come in so it will be a little easier. I am very proud of you for finding a solution and being so mature about your responsibilities. I'm going to tell your father about this when he comes home. He is going to be so happy and proud of you".

▶ **HOW TO USE CPS APPROACH TO TEACH LANGUAGE PROCESSING SKILLS:**

Many ADHD children do not have the language to express their feelings. They don't know how to use the words to express happiness, sadness, frustration, etc. With a younger child, a parent can review the child's daily events and try to identify situations where dealing with feelings was a dominant theme. A good time for this might be just before bedtime.

Mother: "Ben, you remember this afternoon at the playground you were playing with the ball when another boy took it away from you. You got so upset and were looking for me. I took the ball from the boy and gave it back to you."

Ben:" I remember. I couldn't find you."

Mother: "At the time you were looking for me and couldn't find me. You were frustrated."

Ben: "But after I found you and you took the ball away from him, I was ok."

Mother: "Yes, first you were frustrated and then you were happy to get the ball back."

This kind of discussion before bedtime needs to be done daily if possible. It only takes a few minutes but makes the child's feelings more concrete and clear in his mind. This is a good way to coach the child not only in new language skills, but also in reviewing events of the day.

For example:

Ellen and her mother were visiting her grandmother when Ellen's father called. After Ellen's mother finished the conversation with her husband, she gave the phone to Ellen. The call disconnected and Ellen began to cry.

Mother: "Ellen, you are so upset."

Ellen: (continues to cry.)

Mother: "Did your father say anything that upset you?"

Ellen: (continues to cry) "No."

Mother: "Are you frustrated that you could not talk with your father."

Ellen: "Yes."

Mother: "You feel frustrated."

Ellen: "Yes."

Mother: "Tell me what you would like to do."

Ellen: "I want to talk to my father."

Mother: "Would you like for me to dial your father so you can finish your conversation?"

Ellen: "Yes"

Mother: "Tell me what you would like for me to do."

Ellen: (stops crying) "Can you call my father back?"

Mother: "I will call him now. You could have asked me much earlier to call your father. This would have stopped you from feeling so frustrated."

This event needs to be reviewed by the mother again before Ellen goes to sleep. It will help her integrate the feeling of frustration into her lexicon of emotions and enhance her ability to express herself and improve her language skills. Reviewing the event further ingrains the thought process. It is often very effective for parents to point out to their child behavior they observe in others so that they can learn to express themselves with the proper words. "See how frustrated Sarah is when she can't untie the knot? When she gets so upset, she is not able to think how to solve even a simple problem."

When a situation arises where you can teach your child from the unproductive behavior of other children it is beneficial because he is calm at the time and not involved. Later when he behaves in a similar unproductive manner, you can remind your child how his friend was not able to accomplish his goal because he was so frustrated and was unable to think straight. This is a very effective way to turn simple conversations and life experiences into parental coaching.

► **HOW TO USE CPS TO TEACH EMOTIONAL REGULATION SKILLS:**

The need to teach a child to separate his emotional reaction from a particular problem so that he can think clearly and look for a solution to solve the problem can be accomplished with CPS. Empathy helps a child calm down and encourages a better exchange with parents. Since many children fail to recognize and articulate their moods, using CPS can help them admit depression or anxiety.

For example:

Parent: "You are in a bad mood lately."

Child: "Who told you that?"

Parent: "You have been very cranky and unhappy."

Child: How can you tell I'm cranky?

Parent: "Whenever we talk to you or ask you anything, you get upset. Do you know why?"

Child: "No."

Parents: "I remember on Monday when you returned from school that you looked upset".

Child: "I get upset in school."

Parent: "You get upset in school."

Child: "It was after school when I stayed to play with some of the children and we got into a fight".

Parent: "You got into a fight with one of the children."

Child: "He told me that I do not play fast enough when I get the ball. I told him he is stupid and doesn't even know how to play the game. My friend stopped the game and said that he will never play with me or even talk to me anymore."

Parent: "Your friend said he will not play or talk to you any more."

Child: "He also said that he will ask all the others friends in the class not to talk to me".

Parent: "Did the other friends stop talking to you?"

Child: "No, only he did."

Parent: "So for the last two days, you have been upset because of this."

Child: "Yes."

Parent: "My worry is that because of this fight with your friend, you have been in a bad mood at home too and that upsets everybody in the house. Let's think together how you can deal with your relationship with your friend at school and how to be in a better mood at home. Any suggestions?"

Child: "No"

Parent: "When you brother gets into a fight with one of his friends in school, he told him the next day that he did not mean to hurt his feelings. You think you could try this solution?"

Child: "Maybe I will try tomorrow".

Parent: "Just remember, even if this doesn't work, we can find a solution together. We all love you a lot. Let's talk about it tomorrow after you return from school."

Child: "Ok."

► HOW TO USE CPS APPROACH TO TEACH COGNITIVE FLEXIBILITY SKILLS:

Many children with lagging cognitive flexibility skills tend to approach the world in a literal rigid manner. To teach these children to approach problem solving in a more flexible way requires practice over a long time.

Cognitive flexibility requires patience and persistence just like a beginner cannot play a great game of tennis without practicing diligently. Using CPS will expose ADHD children to flexible thinking and train them to examine all possible solutions. Eventually this subtle coaching instills more flexible thinking. These are life skills; not just for young children.

Mother: "I don't think you will be able to play outside today because it's raining".

Child: "You told me that during vacation I can play outside every day".

Mother: "Yes I did, but today it is raining so hard that you can not be outside".

Child: "I'm going out because you said I could every day".

Mother: "You know no other kids will be playing outside".

Child: "I don't care. I want to go outside".

Mother: "Can you think of other activities you would like to do"?

Child: "No".

Mother: "The last time it was raining, I remember you played with your video games and once you made a tent in your room with a cardboard box. What about something like that"?

Child: "Maybe but when it stops raining I want to go outside".

Mother: "I can agree with that."

It will require many such exchanges with a child to teach him to become more flexible in his thinking and actions. Facing new situations will cause anxiety, but pointing out different options to deal with new problems will help the child to consider extending his rigid range of solutions. Most black and white thinkers tend to overreact to minor failures. Statements like: "I am stupid;" "Nobody likes me;" "I'll never be able to do that;" are commonly heard when they feel frustrated.

Child: "I'm stupid."

Mother: "You often say you are stupid."

Child: "I am."

Mother: "I think you're pretty smart so I don't know why you say that"

Child: "I never finish my homework on time and all the other kids do."

Mother: "It takes you longer to do your homework and sometimes you make mistakes because you try to finish too quickly. That's why we are working to be more organized and you are improving all the time."

Child: "I still think I'm stupid."

Mother: "There are many activities where you are very good and not slow at all."

Child: "What do you mean?"

Mother: "Well, what about drawing? And what about how quickly you can put puzzles together. And what about being one of the fastest kids in your class."

Child: Silent

Mother: "It's hard to believe that a stupid kid can be so good at so many things."

Always challenge negative thoughts and replace them with a more positive image. You do not want your child to incorporate into his opinion of himself negative traits.

▶ **HOW TO USE CPS APPROACH TO TEACH SOCIAL SKILLS:**

Many social skills can be coached by reviewing events using CPS to develop adaptive responses. Make sure your child sees the connection between his newly acquired skills and the results of his actions. Failing to recognize how one's behavior is perceived by others or failure to take another person's perspective into account are two major weaknesses that prevent the ADHD from feeling comfortable in a social setting.

For example:

Parent: "You called Max a little girl."

Child: "I did not".

Parent: "I wonder why you did that."

Child: "If I did, I thought it was funny."

Mother: "Max didn't think it was funny and he left to play with someone else. I don't think he'll want to come here to play with you if you make him feel bad."

Child: "I don't care."

Mother: "I think that sometimes you say things before you think and you don't realize that you have hurt someone's feelings."

Child: "I don't want to talk about it."

Mother: "Maybe we will talk about it later. You will miss playing with Max."

Developing new social skills will take time. One discussion on the subject will not change behavior. This maladaptive behavior served the child for a long time, so it is not realistic to expect a rapid change overnight. Parents need to keep working on CPS to train and develop all cognitive skills. The child will be much more open and receptive to discuss solutions and follow plans that he took a part in developing. Discussing the problems with the child improves communication and creates trust between the parent and the child.

► **IMPORTANT POINTS TO REMEMBER:**

- The success of the CPS method is based on the equal participation of the child and the parent.
- Make sure your child is able to express and clearly define his concerns, needs, and worries.

- Express your concerns and wishes so that by the end of the first step, the concerns of both parent and child will be 'on the table.'
- Invite your child to 'brainstorm' with you in exploring all possible solutions.
- Choose the best solution to resolve the issue at hand. The solution must be realistic and address both concerns.
- Some solutions to serious problems can be found only by applying a gradual approach.
- After a week or ten days, review with your child how well the solution you both found together has been executed.
- Empathy and unconditional love will create a calmer atmosphere and go a long way, even before the initial attempt to resolve the problem has begun.
- Not all ADHD children will show deficiencies in all 5 domains of thinking skills.

Chapter 9

BRAIN EXERCISE THERAPY (BET)

▶ **FOR OPTIMUM BRAIN FUNCTION:**

The results achieved with BET were so surprising that few researchers had even theorized that brain exercises might work or have a spill-over effect on functions seemingly totally unrelated to the part of the brain being stimulated. For example, brain exercises to improve the sense of touch resulted in an improvement in auditory function as well! It is as if this stimulation removed a mental block that allowing for numerous mental functions to improve.

All activities that involve exercising the brain, enhancing the connections between neurons and developing memory, as long as there is always increased difficulty, are extremely helpful to children with ADHD. Good-for-everyone mental and physical exercises are the most effective way to make permanent changes in brain function. It is important to emphasize that these exercises need to be intense and a part of the every day routine in order for the child to become proficient. The more sophisticated the exercises, the greater the improvement. And one more thing: Make the whole experience fun and follow with lots of praise.

Adolescents and adults can also take charge of strengthening their minds with vigorous thinking, memory, and physical exercises. Treatment will be discussed in detail in this book.

▶ WHY DO THINKING EXERCISES ENHANCE MENTAL ABILITIES?

This new therapy can be used in all individuals with symptoms of ADHD and is based on the following known facts:

(1) The ADHD brain shows a lack of full development in specific areas responsible for cognitive functioning. The main problem is that the neurotransmitters, for a variety of reasons, are not able to stimulate a full response.

Impulsivity results because the center in charge of *inhibiting* actions sends a very weak signal. The child just goes with his first urge whether it's chasing a ball into the street, blurting out an abrasive comment, or wandering away from his parents. When frustrated or angry, he is unable to think clearly or cope effectively. Furthermore, when he does make a mistake, he usually doesn't learn from it when faced with a similar situation. It may be because he acts so impulsively he never refers to the past. It might be that the signal recording the pain of the first mistake is not fully imprinted in the memory. Whatever theory is correct, the end result is the same: poor impulse control.

(2) The brain can change, grow and become more sophisticated with practice, training and active exercises that impact cognitive areas of the brain. What makes the brain work more effectively is the number of neuronal connections; the more neurons are stimulated, the more they put out additional dendrite connections to neighboring neurons to re-enforce that particular behavior or function. *Neurons that fire together, wire together.*

This is the key to correcting ADHD symptoms. Even if you have insufficient neurotransmitters at each synapse, if you have more synapses supporting the same function, you have essentially raised the level of the neurotransmitter for that specific function.

These changes, unlike any other form of therapy, can be permanent. Just like learning to ride a bicycle, the skill may need a little "polishing" from time to time but you never really forget it. That means the organization of the cerebral cortex can change substantially and actually grow as a result of practice, training and experiences! Isn't it great that a treatment that is completely natural, healthy and can enhance mental abilities will at the same time diminish and finally eliminate ADHD symptoms.

Doing brain exercises that are tailor-made to develop the missing skills is a process of training the brain in specific tasks to impact certain functions of the brain. These changes in the brain will lead to improved concentration, better impulse control and a reduction in hyperactivity. When these exercises are done properly, most ADHD individuals can reduce or eliminate medication and their brain function will be enhanced by increasing the number of neuronal connections and the amount of neurotransmitter present. Since stimulating the brain does indeed make it grow, brain training can lead to full recovery from ADHD symptoms. You can look at it as gymnastics for the brain. There are no limits to the benefits of stimulating and exercising the brain. The brain is constantly adapting itself as a result of learning something new and learning how to learn.

▶ HOW DOES BET WORK?

Exercising the brain with new ways of thinking creates more sophisticated neural pathways for problem solving and acquiring new skills. Brain stimulation recruits hundreds of thousands of nerve cells to develop the missing skills. The capacity of the brain to show this amazing plasticity will result in major improvement in thinking, perception and memory. One needs to keep in mind that real cognitive changes will begin to be noticed only after 50–70 intensive hours of BET. You can not develop muscles after one visit to a sports club; the same applies to BET.

Is your child interested in juggling or magic tricks? Great

brain exercise! *To benefit, the child must master the techniques.* Strategizing, thinking ahead, quick reflexes are all skills that support brain exercise and "spill over" into other problem solving realms.

The areas of the brain responsible for specific tasks, referred to as 'brain maps', vary in size and borders from person to person. Brain maps are influenced by events and actions taken by each individual over the course of a lifetime. After proper treatment, the nervous system can show as much as a 25% increase in the size of specific brain maps associated with the underlying cognitive deficit. These more powerful, more sophisticated neuronal connections will allow the individual to retain more information as well as improve the capacity for learning.

Strengthening a specific function with targeted brain exercises is a type of "cross-training." Children, who were trained to detect very fast vibrations on their skin lasting only 75 milliseconds, could detect 75 millisecond *sounds* as well.

▶ **IS BRAIN PLASTICITY LIMITED BY AGE?**

No. Most neurons show plasticity throughout life with the proper stimulation and exercises. "Use it or lose it" was never more true than it is in the case of brain functioning. However, in the young brain, the number of connections among neurons is about 50% greater than among adult brains. This may explain why children can learn new skills, such as languages, more easily than adolescents or adults. After prolonged treatment, a 5% increase in the weight of the cerebral cortex can be measured. That may not seem like much, but when you are talking about neurons, i.e. "grey matter", it represents hundreds of millions of new neuronal connections. Developing all types of thinking and memory skills increase the number of branches among neurons and this leads to an increase in the size, weight and sophistication of the brain.

The brain is constantly adapting itself as a result of new

learning. The newly formed structures then enhance the learning process in a virtuous feedback.

▶ **DOES THE NERVOUS SYSTEM IN ADHD WORK DIFFERENTLY?**

No. The brain works the same with or without ADHD.

The axon that first picks up the signal starts the process of transporting a message to the dendrite of the neighboring neuron much like an electrical impulse along a conductive wire. Two types of signals, inhibitory and stimulatory, can be received by the neurons. As soon as an electrical signal reaches the end of the axon, it stimulates the release of neurotransmitters from the dendrite of the neurons. Dopamine and other neurotransmitters are the stimulants for conduction of cognitive impulses. In a resting situation, dopamine is stored in tiny sacs in the nerve cell and, when stimulated, is released into the synapse or space between the axon and the neighboring dendrite. The neurons do not physically touch each other. *Effective transmission in that space is critical to neuronal function and here is where the deficiency is found in* ADHD *cases.* There is not enough active neurotransmitter (dopamine) to stimulate a complete response. Ritalin temporarily increases the amount of free dopamine in the synapse and brings the conductivity back to normal. BET increases the number and complexity of synapses to achieve normal levels of free dopamine.

▶ **THE CENTRAL NERVOUS SYSTEM WITH AND WITHOUT ADHD:**

Some areas of the ADHD brain are slightly smaller and have less neurons for the transfer of impulses. In addition, ADHD individuals have less of the neurotransmitter in the neuronal synapse.

That means the response to any stimulation will be weak and incomplete. This explains why most ADHD children seem to have poor concentration and poor utilization of working memory to help them formulate proper decisions. If there is not enough do-pamine available for a full response, there is very little likelihood of impulse control. Without an effective inhibitory mechanism, thoughtless comments, lack of planning, and impulsive behavior are the inevitable consequences. Doing BET for at least 45 minutes each day for six days coupled with CPS will bring real change in the level of dopamine in the brain which will manifest itself in better thinking skills, more reflective thought processes and greater organization.

▶ WHY IS IT SO HARD TO BREAK BAD HABITS?

When we learn a bad habit, a pathway is created in the brain. The more we repeat this behavior, the stronger and more entrenched it will become. We can look at neural pathway as digging microscopic trenches. Each re-enforcement digs the trench a little bit deeper each time. Using the same pathway over and over again makes it much harder to forge a new pathway. When we learn a good or bad habit, there is a physical change in the neuronal mechanism in the brain. Each time we repeat this behavior, the pathway becomes more dedicated to this behavior. Anytime we try to use new behavior, the brain will resist the attempt to forge a new pathway. That is why the breaking of old habits is so difficult. You can also apply the same principles to a sense of taste. Children that are constantly given sweets will have difficulty appreciating other tastes and will even resist them. Brain exercises stimulate neurons to become more selective, more efficient and learn to process information more efficiently and faster. Faster neurons lead to quick thinking and stronger signals that will improve memory and have a greater impact on all brain activities. What we want to develop is good productive thinking habits. The power of habits was expressed centuries before we understood brain function: "The beginning of a habit is like an invisible thread, but every time we repeat the act, we strengthen the strand, add to it another filament, until it becomes a great cable and binds us irrevocably in thought and act." That is why the creation of productive habits such as organizational skills and problem solving abilities so clearly define the quality and efficiency of our life.

▶ **WHAT IS A TYPICAL BET EXPERIENCE FOR CHILDREN?**

The most important thing is to make the exercise fun. If the exercise is not enjoyable, the child will not stick with it. You should focus on your child's interests and abilities. Some children need help to discover activities they really like. Keep trying.

Any single BET is not enough. Remember, the activity must be intense and daily.

You want the child to develop expertise. Keep in mind that the goal is to literally re-enforce neuronal connections and this may take several months to establish. The more stimulation, the better the results. We all derive great pleasure from developing talent and abilities. Your child will too.

(1) What is an interest of your child? Use it. For example, children often develop intense interests. If they are fascinated with cats or dogs, buy books that discuss the different types and their names. For example, reward your child for learning the order of events in the Bible by heart. Then increase the complexity, i.e. does this event come before or after another specific event, etc. The child can learn the team jersey numbers and statistics of his favorite team players. A list of the national championship teams in the last 50 years can be memorized. Then ask him to remember who was the national champion in 1955 or who was most valuable player.

(2) Find educational video games where the player cannot move to the next level without first mastering the prior level. Use those with an educational purpose that involves planning and strategy.

(3) Physical endeavors such as martial arts develop focus, discipline, concentration as well as physical abilities.

(4) Expose your child to computers. There are many educational computer games and lessons to improve memory, strategic planning and thinking skills. Pajama Sam is very good for young children.

(5) Encourage his memory skills with poems, songs and puzzles. Always increase the level of complexity.

(6) Memory exercises are good for all ages. The key for effective memory exercises is to focus on areas of interest. Children typically develop intense interests. For example, if your child is fascinated with cats or horses, encourage him to learn the names of all the different species.

When his interests change, repeat the process.

(7) Teach your child to play chess. It's great for strategy, working memory, planning and delayed gratification.

(8) Rummikub is effective game to enhance memory and planning and a great activity for the family to do together.

(9) Magic tricks involve strategy, planning ahead, good reflexes.

Be creative and try to think of activities that encourage brain development in areas of concentration, memory and problem solving. Make vigorous exercise fun, encourage sports and balance exercises and institute physical exercise as a part of family activities. Remember to lavish praise for a job well done.

(10) To strengthen visual memory, teach your child to recognize the shapes of the letters of a foreign language. Tracing the letters is an excellent exercise. You can choose Greek, Persian, Russian or English letters and he can learn to write the letters and their position in the order of the alphabet. This can be a part of learning a second language. After the task of learning the letters and recognizing the proper order, ask him to recognize the letters by naming the number of the letter in the order of the ABCs. The next level is to ask him to recognize certain letters based on their position. For example, which is the fifth letter before 'o'.

(11) I cannot emphasize enough how beneficial it is for your

ADHD child to learn a second language. This can be encouraged by the use of foreign language cartoons on TV, sending your child to a kindergarten where another language is spoken or with tutoring or a babysitter that can speak a different language, etc. It is so easy for a child to learn a second or third language in childhood and so very difficult to learn as an adult. It has been shown that learning additional languages improves memory, math skills, abstract learning and reading in all children, not just ADHD.

▶ **WHAT ARE SOME OF THE PRINCIPLES OF BET?**

Many activities can contribute to enhancement of brain functions. BET will improve memory, thinking skills, impulsivity, language skills and concentration to mention a few of the benefits to the brain. Each exercise will have to be built according to the level of difficulties beginning at a very simple level. The goal is to move from level to level so that the child will experience a sense of accomplishment with each new challenge. At the completion of each level, give your child a special reward. This reward is crucial to the success of BET. Each time the child is rewarded for accomplishment, his brain secretes a substance which helps consolidate the changes developed in the neuronal pathways, i.e. entrenches the ski path. Rewards are a natural way to encourage use of these exercises.

Since brain enhancement is related to the length of time you exercise it, the recommendation for a typical brain workout is at least 45 minutes to an hour a day, five days a week for six to eight weeks. Make sure the entire experience will be fun for your child and not viewed as a chore. You will find that if your child is really passionate about an activity, you will not have much trouble getting him involved.

Which type of BET improves concentration?

As a consultant to a Russian clinic in Moscow, I was exposed to specific brain exercises that helped to improve concentration.

These exercises required the use of pencils held in both hands to draw simultaneously the same geometrical form. You could start by drawing different sizes of squares on both sheets of paper. Also drawing the same size on both papers and gradually increase the size of the square set 4 sizes. Once you master drawing 4 different sizes of squares, you start drawing circles in different sizes and then triangles. The second stage you try to draw simultaneously different geometric forms using both hands, i.e. a triangle with one hand and a circle with the other.. You start by drawing squares with one hand while drawing a triangle with the other. The exercise is then done again after switching hands.

For this exercise to have a real impact, they have to be done for no less than 20 minutes, six days a week. It is also interesting to note that, even today, Russian education holds in high esteem good penmanship and students are expected to practice until perfect. Along the same vein, a great deal more memory work is used in Russian classes. In contrast, we seem to find ways to use our memory less rather than more with Power Point presentations, Blackberries and other memory crutches.

▶ **WHICH OTHER TYPES OF BET WILL STIMULATE NEURONAL GROWTH?**

Tracing complex lines will improve small muscle control in the hand as well improve concentration and focus. You can use Chinese letters or other symbols.

Memory exercises have other positive influences on brain function as well as small hand muscle control. Poems or new vocabulary will improve auditory memory. All listening exercises will improve concentration and enhance the ability to follow instructions. You can create you own memory exercises. Speaking in a soft voice will encourage your child to listen closely.

Building a rich vocabulary and using the new words in every day conversations is a wonderful exercise with many benefits.

Matching games to put together the new words with their meaning makes it fun.

► **CAN YOU IMPROVE THE THINKING PROCESS?**

Yes. On average, most children can remember five to seven digits or items. Often ADHD children can usually remember only three or four. *These poor memory skills cause poor use of spoken language and this leads to slow thinking.* This undeveloped skill can be treated with BET. Each day ask your child to write down the best part of his day during school and then read it together. On alternate days, ask him to write about two conflicts he faced.

Review together how he resolved the conflict and point out each time alternative ways to resolve the same problem. Don't forget to praise his efforts. On alternative days, present your child with one or two problems and let him try to find solutions to these problems. Here the key is to reward your child with proper recognition for his attempt to resolve the problem. The reward will contribute as much as finding the solution.

Once again, building vocabulary increases memory, develops thinking skills and enhances concentration. Be sure to include lots of words that express the whole range of human emotion.

► **WHAT ARE THE BENEFITS TO TEACHING MY CHILD NEW SKILLS?**

This is the most effective way to lead to neuronal growth and brain changes. New skills can include such challenges as learning a musical instrument, dancing, judo, gymnastics, drawing, painting and skating because all are very useful skills for BET. Any organized sports activities will bring about similar results. In addition to new skills, your child will be doing activities persistently and moving up the ladder of success and accomplishment. Here you can develop your own system of reward and find the activities that compliment your child's interests and talents.

You can do a project together such as building an airplane

model or some other structure out of matches. Once again, the key to success with BET is persistence and regular stimulation every day. To make the activity more fun, you may ask more family members to participate. Teaching your child to play chess may be the most rewarding. In addition to learning how to strategize, consider options and plan for the future, chess players will develop certain patterns of play that they will use. Chess masters store up to 50,000 patterns in their memory.

▶ CAN EXERCISE GENERATE NEW BRAIN CELLS?

Yes. Physical exercise is one of the main and most important pillars of treatment. Aerobics is beneficial for everyone; for the ADHD brain, it is essential. If possible, include sports such as martial arts for discipline, balance, quicker reflexes and concentration but any kind of aerobic exercise has a very positive impact on the ADHD brain. Scientists at Columbia University compared MRI scans of those who exercise regularly with those who don't. Those who exercise regularly had more blood flow to the hippocampus; a critical structure for memory. This increase in blood flow reflects an increase in brain cells. Scientists gave the subjects a set of cognitive tests and found that the more physically fit the person was, the better he would perform on memory tests. For exercise to be effective, the child needs to be involved in vigorous exercise for at least 20 minutes five times a week.

▶ CAN VIDEO GAMES IMPROVE BRAIN FUNCTIONING?

Yes. Many parents will express disbelief that some video games can sharpen thinking, improve social skills, perception and general brain functioning. Pre-school age video game "Pajama Sam"is an example that serves as a good brain exercise. Video games can be mentally enriching by improving the system of thinking, persistence, patience, concentration, willingness to delay gratification and learning to prioritize resources. As with just about anything else in this world, video games can be used or abused.

University of California research shows that the brain consumes a great deal of energy doing video games which indicates the high level of work the brain does while playing. A new book by John Back, professor at Harvard Medical School, looks at three types of professionals: hardcore game players, occasional game players and non-game players. Those who played regularly turned out to be more sociable, more confident and able to solve problems much more creatively and easily than non-game players. Many video games serve the goals of BET as they do not allow progress to a higher level of play without reaching a certain level of expertise. Just be selective, use common sense and choose those games that serve to stimulate the parts of the brain where skills are lagging. For example, games that resemble chess or chess itself, are excellent. The player must strategize, reflect on the past and the consequences of future moves and concentrate and focus in order to succeed in moving to the next level of skill. This is a great way to make brain exercises fun and is suitable for all ages.

Most video games will reward for successful accomplishment at each level of the game. Video games are also non-judgmental; the child does not have to face teasing or failure in front of others. Game playing triggers dopamine release in the brain as well, but one needs to limit the playing of video games to prevent preoccupation with this type of exercise only. You want your child to be well-rounded so that no single activity is excessive. You want to strike a balance between developing real expertise but not having one activity dominate all others.

▶ **HOW IMPORTANT IS BET IN THE TREATMENT OF ADHD?**

This new model of therapy is crucial in treating and correcting ADHD symptoms. We discussed several types of brain exercises but you can create your own training exercises with your child tailored to his particular interests. You need to be flexible and use your imagination and knowledge of your child to find the most enjoyable exercise for your child. This program will not be effective unless implemented at least five days a week. We hope your child will develop a real love and passion for his chosen activities. In most cases, you can begin to see some improvement with BET in three months and the improvement is proportional to the level of skill that is acquired. Activities such as sports, exercise, etc. should be continued throughout life for a healthy body and mind.

► **IMPORTANT POINTS TO REMEMBER:**

- BET is one of the most effective ways to treat ADHD children.
- New brain skills will develop as a result of BET.
- BET needs to be practiced in as many different activities as the child enjoys five days a week for 12 weeks before you can expect to see results.
- There are several categories of BET that can be used for practice.
- Auditory and visual BET will improve many brain functions.
- Vigorous exercise will generate new connections among neurons and improve memory.
- Video games can sharpen thinking processes, improve social skills and develop problem solving capabilities. As with everything else, nothing should be done in *excess* and games must be chosen carefully.
- Learning a new language will enhance memory, abstract learning and even math skills as well as reduce the symptoms of ADHD.
- BET capitalizes on the natural adaptability and development of mental abilities. Any skill is undeveloped until you decide to master it.

Chapter 10

MULTI-DISCIPLINARY METHOD TO STIMULATE BRAIN GROWTH

Every activity that stimulates brain growth in children is also effective in teenagers and adults. Clearly *only* jogging or *only* memory exercises is inadequate for the dramatic results that are possible with full implementation of all strategies. However, it is accurate to say that each makes a contribution.

A multi-disciplinary approach will not only contribute to a happier, more confident child but also build a more flexible sophisticated brain, enhances social skills and memory development.

▶ **WHAT IS THE SQ3R METHOD TO IMPROVE MEMORY?**

A good strategy to improve concentration and develop effective memory and recall is by using the SQ3R method: Survey, Question, Read, Recite and Review. First step is to give your child an overview of the new material. Second, ask him questions about the material. The child will then have a better understanding of the new topic when he reads about it. Third, encourage him to speak about what he just read. And finally, review the material later. This will help the child retain the information. ADHD children who know how to employ this method will feel less overwhelmed and more importantly, this tool will help him concentrate better because he will have a consistent guideline to help him study new material.

▶ **WHY IS REWARD VERY IMPORTANT TO THE BRAIN EXERCISE PROGRAM?**

Although you will try to make brain exercises fun and interesting, some of the activities may need to be monotonous to develop concentration under more difficult circumstances. By giving a reward for a job well done at the end of each practice session, you will enhance motivation and interest and give your child a feeling of accomplishment. A reward given for serious effort will reassure and inspire greater effort in the future. This can be tied to receiving an allowance. You can use tokens or poker chips to be accumulated during the week and paid out in the form of an allowance.

Accomplishment needs praise and encouragement. *Reward causes secretion of dopamine in neuronal synapses to "cement" the memory or skill.*

▶ **CAN YOU PLAY GAMES THAT WILL IMPROVE CONCENTRATION?**

Yes. Any card game can be used that involves memory, concentration and focus.

You could create your own cards and games. You could design ten cards with colors, shapes, pictures, etc., review the order with your child and ask him to repeat the order. This game can easily be made more complex. You can focus on the numbers, then on the numbers and colors.

You can create mazes to be conquered and steadily increase their complexity.

A maze of "let's go to the beach as quickly as possible" or the typical mouse and cheese can be used. It's easy to create your own or you will find them in many children's magazines and on the internet.

The possibilities are endless and you can incorporate your child's interests.

A maze of "help the puppy find his way home" would appeal to a dog lover. You can simply write 120 letters in ten rows of 12 letters in each row. Ask your child to identify as many words as possible or how many r's are in the line up for a younger child.

▶ DO ALTERNATIVE TREATMENTS WORK?

If by "alternative treatment" you mean herbal remedies or other holistic remedies that claim to treat ADHD, there is not a shred of unbiased scientific evidence that they are effective. Further, there is no independent agency responsible for checking the contents for contaminants such as heavy metals or pesticides or even to verify that the contents are the same as the label. Occasionally there will be a scientific study which will identify side effects of some popular herbal treatment to boost the immune system or some other unsubstantiated claim. These side effects are often not benign such as decreased fertility. Insist of evidence of effectiveness before you spend your hard-earned money on something totally ineffective and possibly harmful.

▶ WHAT ARE THE MOST COMMON ALTERNATIVE TREATMENTS FOR ADHD?

Many parents are reluctant to medicate their loved ones. Recent studies show that about 80% of patients that start medication for treatment of ADHD quit after a year. More than 50% of American families who receive treatment for ADHD by physicians also use complimentary therapies or modify their lifestyle. The most commonly used alternative therapies for ADHD are dietary changes and dietary supplements. Lifestyle changes that parents can use with considerable positive results include different types of exercise and outdoor activities.

► CAN A PARENT HELP THEIR CHILD'S VISION AND THINKING SKILLS?

Yes. For example, you can buy a large city map and teach your child to read a map. Once he is familiar with the map of his town, you can ask him to locate specific places to find the shortest route from one location to another. You can also use outings in town to help develop a sense of direction by encouraging him to remember the map and help you find certain locations. Every outing with your child should be full of questions to encourage him to think. When he makes a mistake in direction, encourage him to find a solution to being "lost" and point out that most problems have several solutions. Let your child help in planning future trips and finding the shortest way to your destination.

Children need to learn math tables so be preemptive. Encourage recitation of math tables that are age appropriate. This will have the added benefit of helping him perform in school.

You can draw any geometric figure. Ask your child to trace this figure, then to copy it by drawing it with his right hand and then his left hand and finally from memory.

Repeat this game daily using different geometric shapes. You can gradually increase the complexity of the shapes and the speed with which the drawings are done.

Use a paragraph in a magazine and ask your child to circle all the B's. Repeat for several days using different letters. Find an action filled picture, show it to your child and ask him to study the details for a few minutes. Then ask him questions such as how many buildings are in the picture, how many people, what is the color of…, etc.

Use music to increase sensitivity to sounds. Play your child's favorite song. Lower the volume until it is barely audible. Very slowly turn up the volume to the point where your child can clearly understand the words. You can make the game more difficult by playing a child's song that he is not so familiar with and ask him to repeat the words at a very low volume. This improves concentration and hearing. Ask your child to identify different noises in and around the house. Ask him to report and describe new sounds on a regular basis.

When you are working in the kitchen you can ask your child to identify different smells with his eyes closed such as a flower, onion, pepper, soap, different food cooking, etc. You could make a simple display of different substances with distinctive smells such as spices and ask him to identify them with his eyes closed.

► ARE THERE ADDITIONAL WAYS TO IMPROVE THINKING SKILLS?

You can present your child with a problem to solve. "What if a tiger escaped from the zoo." "What if a child on the playground does not let you play with his ball?" "What if your friend is mad at you?" "What are different ways to say you're sorry?"

"What would he take with him if he was an astronaut on his way to the moon?"

Ask your child to present each day at least two problems he was facing and let him review how he handled the problems.

You can plan an association game by asking your child to match pairs of pictures in a set of twenty pictures such as fish and water, trees and flowers. You can steadily make the associations less obvious and more sophisticated.

You can have your child recite the alphabet and a word associated with each letter. Many board games such as scrabble, puzzles, checkers, dominoes and chess are examples of games that are mentally stimulating.

Design mazes or connect-the-dots puzzles.

▸ IS VIGOROUS EXERCISE EFFECTIVE?

Yes, there is an improvement in the symptoms of ADHD with exercise. Regular aerobic exercise programs not only improve symptoms and modify behavior of the child or teen, but also promote brain development. Stephen C. Putnam in his book "Nurturing your ADHD Child with Exercise: Nature's Ritalin for the Marathon Mind", promotes the idea of exercise as an alternative treatment for ADHD. Putnam believes that aerobic exercise has an effect on the brain that is similar to Ritalin and other psycho-stimulants. A targeted exercise program can have a major impact on symptoms. Aerobic exercise increases levels of neurotransmitters (dopamine, serotonin and norepinephrine), improving emotional stability, focus, mental alertness and calm. The intensity, duration and frequency of the aerobic exercise determine the degree of change in the brain. To get the most benefit from exercise you need to incorporate brain exercises daily and achieve real skill and endurance. Sports or activities that involved strategy and planning or an exercise program using dance moves or more sophisticated coordination are superior.

Charles Hillman from the University of Illinois reports in his book that vigorous aerobic exercise coaxes the human brain into growing new nerve cells; a phenomenon that for decades has been considered impossible.

With regular exercise, nerve cells branch out, join together and communicate with each other in new ways that are the critical to new learning processes. In addition the brain is washed with increased oxygen and nutrients, growth factors and neural elements. Hillman reports that exercise improves not just executive function like planning, organization and decision-making, but also math, reading, and logical thinking. Recent experiments at schools in Naperville, Illinois have also proven very interesting. Students with poor verbal skills who take physical education immediately before a reading class showed improved performance within a few months, as based on their report cards.

Even random exercise has a positive effect. BET magnifies this positive development. Every activity mastered by the child lays down new neuronal pathways which results in a quicker more flexible cortex. Aerobic exercise done before doing homework improves concentration, memory and focus. Hopefully, someday this will be also incorporated into the school system to improve school performance.

▶ WHAT KINDS OF EXERCISE PROGRAMS GET RESULTS?

Significant improvement in behavior can be achieved with about a half hour of intense exercise five days a week. This can include a reduction in oppositional defiance and aggressive behavior as well as improvement in concentration and focus.

There are a few aerobic exercises that can be incorporated into your child's daily program: At least 20 minutes of vigorous exercise at one time and 10 minutes of moderate intensity; Hiking, walking at speeds of 10 min/km, bicycling at rate of 15 km/hr, swimming, jump rope, tap or jazz dancing, soccer, basketball etc. If a parent can make the exercise effort a family affair, that's even better. I can't remember who first noted: "Families that play together, stay together." Everyone will benefit. Having a positive attitude and shared interests encourage the child to follow the program and stick with it.

▶ WHAT IS THE EFFECT OF BALANCE THERAPY?

Another type of exercise that has a positive effect on reducing ADHD symptoms is balance therapy. Here some of the aerobic exercise is supplemented with balance exercises that improve the relationship between different functional areas of the brain. Often people with ADHD also have a poor sense of balance. Even if balance is not impaired, these exercises improve and refine the interaction between cognitive and memory centers of the brain through the use of existing neurons and creates neuro-pathways between these centers that did not exist before. Special exercise programs bring about the interaction of sensory processing with the sensory integration activities. This will help improve the way the brain processes information. Different balance exercises can be started with the help of a physical therapist or by a resourceful parent who can design a program of balance and aerobic exercises, such as ballet and gymnastics. To see an effect, the child will have to be involved five days a week, each time for no less than 20–30 minutes. Parents should incorporate both types of exercise, aerobic and balance- aerobic for when the child returns from school and before he starts his homework, and balance before he goes to bed. There are several well-established programs that recommend balance exercises to stimulate the cerebellum. This small area at the rear of the brain contains 50% of the neurons of the brain and receives 50% of the brain's blood supply. Some researchers suggest that the cerebellum also plays a major role is short term memory, attention, impulse control, thinking and emotion. The cerebellum connects to the frontal lobes which is the reason improvement is quite dramatic in activities that seem unrelated to balance.

Balance exercises increase blood supply to the cerebellum, leading to improved brain function. Any exercise that includes eye-hand coordination, eye movement exercises, ballet or dancing will contribute to cerebellum stimulation. Be creative and build your own program of balance exercises that suits your child's interests. The Dore Program and the Brain Gym pioneered the development of this concept. Regular exercise combined with balance exercises also improve mood, decrease anxiety, improve sleep and raise self-esteem.

Which games of coordination and balance improve brain function?
Teach your child to use both hands for different tasks. The old game of patting the stomach and making horizontal motions

above your head with the other hand is typical. Once this is done easily, then switch tasks to the opposite hand. Practice until task is done quite easily and rapidly. Then increase the complexity by added additional moves.

You can use pictures in old magazines and ask your child to cut out different subjects in the picture, i.e. trees, buildings, people, animals, etc. keeping as close to the lines as possible. Once this task is done well, switch hands. Keep this up until he can do this very well. Always praise his accomplishments.

Buy or make a balance board. After two weeks of daily use for ten minutes, balance will improve. You can improve balance by standing on one foot with eyes closed. Make it a game. Reward improvement.

Juggling can be gradually increased in complexity. Don't let your child get discouraged. When balance and coordination improves, concentration and focus will improve also.

Learning magic tricks combines many complex tasks such as planning ahead, reflexes, coordination, focus and concentration.

At a later stage, you can tie many of these activities together with music and rhythm. You are literally helping the cortex to grow.

Can Yoga and Ballet diminish ADHD symptoms?
Yes. Control studies completed in 2004 proved that after six weeks of biweekly ballet or yoga classes conducted for 30 minutes with a trained instructor and continued daily at home with the parent, diminished many ADHD symptoms significantly.

▸ CAN DIET IMPACT ADHD SYMPTOMS?
There are two primary diets that have been associated with ADHD-like symptom relief.

Feingold Diet: This diet is based on the elimination of 3 groups of synthetic additives and synthetic sweeteners. All synthetic colors, synthetic flavors and all artificial sweeteners such as aspartane and sucrazit are avoided.

A study of 1800 three year olds with hyperactive behavior in England showed significant improvement in behavior with a diet free of preservatives and artificial flavors. When these items were re-introduced, the behavior returned. Based on these studies, schools in Wales banned foods containing additives from school lunches in 2004.

Synthetic additives and sweeteners are not essential ingredients for anyone's diet and some children respond positively after eliminating them. Such a change in diet can do no harm and may, in fact, help your child.

Sugar restriction diet for ADHD: Many studies trying to determine the impact of a sugar-free diet on the behavior of ADHD symptoms have failed to prove a relationship between sugar and an increase or decrease in ADHD symptoms. Sugar contributes to dental cavities and obesity. Even though no relationship has yet been found with ADHD symptoms, empty calories should be minimized.

▶ CAN ALLERGIES CAUSE ADHD-LIKE SYMPTOMS?

Yes. There are many reports of food allergies as a main cause of ADHD-like symptoms. Although this does not apply to true ADHD, just as preservatives and additives can cause similar symptoms, allergies to milk, wheat, corn, cats, dogs, and molds to name a few, can cause ADHD-*like* symptoms in some children. Avoiding allergy triggers can resolve many related problems.

An allergy to milk and milk products can cause 'brain fog'; wheat and corn can cause irritability; molds can cause headaches; and gluten sensitivity is linked to increased risk of other ADHD symptoms. Studies show that a large percentage of children with ADHD symptoms, when referred to a nutrition clinic, improved after their diet was changed. Clearly, these children do not have ADHD but only similar symptoms.

In conclusion, we can state that a diet free of preservatives, allergens and additives can improve ADHD symptoms in some cases. Identify allergies, eliminate junk food as much as possible, and include lots of fruits and vegetables in the daily diet – that's good advice for anyone.

I am always amazed when I hear of parents spreading chocolate or jelly on white bread along with potato chips for their children's lunch. What are they thinking? The effects of what we put in the mouths of our children cannot be overestimated. All children need a nutritious diet for optimum mental and physical development.

► CAN VITAMIN AND MINERAL SUPPLEMENTS CONTROL ADHD SYMPTOMS?

Studies conducted in the past failed to show a contribution of vitamin B-6 (pyridoxine) and vitamin C toward the reduction of ADHD symptoms. No vitamin above daily requirements was found to be useful in treating children with ADHD.

Several reports in the past indicated that mineral deficiencies are more commonly found among children with ADHD. The three most common minerals that parents need to check are iron, zinc and magnesium. One way to give trace minerals is by using unrefined salt or use a multi-vitamin and mineral supplement. Make sure your child eats plenty of fresh fruits and vegetables as well. Stick with whole wheat products and other high nutrient products.

Omega 3 fatty acids and Melatonin:

Children with lower levels of Omega 3 fatty acids seem to have significantly more behavioral problems, temper tantrums and sleep problems than those with higher levels of Omega 3 fatty acids. A typical diet is woefully low in Omega 3.

Studies of children with coordination difficulties show significant improvement in reading, spelling and behavior after three months of treatment with Omega 3 fatty acids. Fatty-acid supplements of 800 mg per day for at least three months may significantly improve reading, spelling and other problems associated with ADHD.

Researchers at the University of Pittsburgh Medical Center recently reported a correlation between higher blood levels of Omega-3 and less impulsive behavior. Taking up to 800 mg per day of Omega-3 is recommended for all children with ADHD since fish oil is very safe and seems to help. You should buy only from a reputable company whose fish oil is not contaminated with heavy metals. If your child will eat fish like salmon, make it a part of his diet. Flax seed has high levels of Omega 3.

It is highly doubtful that Omega 3 by itself will eliminate ADHD symptoms since the real problem lies with a deficiency in neurotransmitters. However, instituting a better diet and optimizing brain nutrients through supplements or naturally is worthwhile.

Melatonin supplements help some ADHD children with sleep problems. Children with ADHD and chronic insomnia who were given 5 mg of melatonin or a placebo showed that there was a significantly improved sleep onset, decreased sleep latency and increased total sleep time.

▶ **IS "GREEN TIME" USEFUL IN THE TREATMENT OF ADHD SYMPTOMS?**

Yes. Children with ADHD should spend some quality time after school hours and weekends outdoors enjoying nature when possible. Studies that appeared in the September issue of the American Journal of Public Health in 2006 pointed out those children that participated in a nationwide study, where each spent 30 minutes to an hour in nature demonstrated a significant reduction in ADHD symptoms. The advantage of outdoor activities was observed among children living in different regions, from rural to large city environments. According to Frances E. Kuo and

Andrea Taylor exposure to nature may help reduce ADHD symptoms. The 400 children in their study participated in a wide range of activities in various locations. Some were indoors and some outdoors in places without much greenery, such as parking lots and downtown areas. Others were in a relatively natural outdoor setting such as yards, parks or tree lined streets. Those who spent time in nature showed a reduction in symptoms.

► **CAN TEACHING YOUR CHILD RELAXATION TECHNIQUES REDUCE SYMPTOMS?**

Yes. One very effective way to reduce your child's stress is to teach him how to relax. Children and teens with ADHD anger easily, lose control and are frequently in conflict. These children can be taught to develop techniques that help them regain control of their emotions. Deep breathing relaxation techniques can dissipate some stress and help children develop coping mechanisms to control emotional outbursts. Teach your child to breathe slowly and deeply before acting or speaking out. Doing relaxation exercises together may turn out to be a wonderful shared activity.

► **WHAT CAN WE DO AS A FAMILY TO REDUCE THE SYMPTOMS OF ADHD?**

Regular and Special Events with ADHD Children:
Mealtime:

One of the most important parts of the day for your child is the family meal. Establish this at least two or three times a week. On nights when the whole family cannot be together, keep the family meal routine on the same schedule if possible. Keeping the same timetable for meals is an important part of the general organizational thinking you want your child to assume. Try to make family meals a regular event. This is an ideal time to share good events of the day and shower praise on the children. This is *not* the time to solve problems!

Many children on medication have poor appetites. Keep this

in mind when you prepare meals. Family meal time is also ideal for developing language skills. You can ask each family member to talk about the best/most interesting/exciting event of their day or ask questions about their activities that will encourage conversation. This is also a great time to include new vocabulary words.

Bed Time:

You must keep regular bedtime routines. A lower level of activity toward bedtime is always a good idea, which is why balancing exercises are recommended. Avoid vigorous exciting activities one hour before bedtime.

Dark and quiet bedrooms help a child relax. No activities should take place in bed other than reading or sleeping. Taking warm baths before going to bed may help your child relax and prepare for sleep. Once in bed, no phone calls or any other distraction should be allowed. Make sure to check all schoolwork before going to bed and to organize clothes for the next day each night.

Special Events with Mother or Father:

Very few activities have a more positive long-term effect on a child than spending special one on one time with his parents. Many adults reflect with pleasure about special time they spent with their mother or father as children. This time is beneficial to everyone, but especially to the ADHD child. Activities can include day trips, going together to a sporting or cultural event, or perhaps enjoying a hobby together. Regular participation of the parents with the child in any area will contribute tremendously to the child's confidence and self-esteem. The ADHD child needs a great deal more feedback and positive re-enforcement. Once a week, review areas of strength and areas for improvement. Praise *first*, suggest improvements last.

Treatment of ADHD can have multiple approaches. In the beginning, medication under the supervision of a physician followed by the CPS and BET approach is very effective. The addition of aerobic and balancing exercises together with Omega 3 fatty acids intake and ruling out allergy triggers should be included. When all of the steps discussed are in place and a few months of positive results are evident, you may talk to your physician about reducing the dose of methylphenidate.

► **IMPORTANT POINTS TO REMEMBER:**

- Brain tissue responds to brain exercises by growing.
- Many parts of the brain can be targeted to improve function.
- Improvement in the function of one specific part of the brain can lead to improved function in other brain areas.
- Memory can be strengthened by such simple strategies as repetition of the information.
- By using the SQ3R method, "Survey, Question, Read, Recite and Review," the child can enhance his memory recall.
- Reward for the completion of each brain exercise is essential to the success of the program.
- Effective brain exercise programs will target all the senses.
- Mix different games during each brain exercise to make the effort fun.
- Keep working on thinking exercises to help your child improve his thinking and language skills as well as emotional regulation.
- Aerobic exercise is very effective in helping to reduce ADHD symptoms, improve memory, social skills and thinking capacity.
- For vigorous exercise to be effective, one needs to exercise at least 30 minutes five days a week.
- Balance therapy seems to have positive effects on ADHD symptoms. To get the full benefit of these types of exercise, they need to be done for 20 minutes, five days a week.
- Diet without chemical additives or artificial sweetener reduces the risk of developing ADHD-like symptoms.

- Omega 3 fatty acids and Melatonin are useful in reducing ADHD-like symptoms.
- Allergies to food such as milk, wheat, corn or certain animals or molds can cause the appearance of ADHD-like symptoms.
- "Green Time"for the ADHD child several times a week for more than 30 minutes was found to be useful in reducing ADHD symptoms.
- Teaching a child with ADHD symptoms to use relaxation techniques can be useful in reducing stress and teaching the child to cope with challenges.
- Work to create family bonding and team efforts through activities enjoyed by the whole family.
- Building vocabulary, learning a new language, etc. have significant benefits, and all children should be encouraged in these endeavors.

Chapter 11

BEHAVIOR THERAPY FOR ADHD

► **WHAT ARE THE PRINCIPLES OF BEHAVIORAL THERAPY?**

There are 3 components to establishing a successful behavioral therapy program at home.

1. Establish a list of target behaviors or tasks a child needs to complete.

Here are a few examples of target behaviors:

At Home:

Brush teeth every morning.
Clean room
Do homework
Complete house chores
Do not fight with siblings
Put toys and games in their place

At School:

Do not answer questions before asked

Do not disturb the class

Remain seated during class

2. Establish a system of reward and punishment to motivate a child to be better behaved and compliant.

Examples of rewards:

    a. New toy or computer game

    b. Privilege to go to a movie

    c. Privilege to go on a trip

    d. Allowance

    e. Concert or sport event

3. Develop a currency system of tokens or points so that rewards and punishments can be recorded and treated appropriately. Each reward should correspond to certain number of points.

Using this kind of program is most effective in managing the behavior of ADHD children between the ages of 4–10, and is most effective in managing certain types of behavior. Some parents complain that once the program ends, many symptoms return. To implement and complete the program, the parents need to spend at least one full week mastering each step before moving to the next. The implementation of Step 1 through 3 lays the foundation for parent-child interaction.

▶ **STEP 1. LEARN TO PAY POSITIVE ATTENTION TO YOUR CHILD:**

Learn to pay positive attention to your child, focusing on his desirable behavior alone. Try to find any opportunity to make positive statements of praise and approval. Statements like: "You are so much fun to play with!" "Terrific move!" and "I'm going to tell your father how much help you were today."

If the child misbehaves, try to overlook it at this stage. If it continues, say you will return to play when he behaves nicely.

Make a point of continuing the praise and positive statements at every opportunity from this point on.

The most effective approval is said immediately. If your child does something well or something thoughtful, make sure he receives praise from you on the spot.

▶ **STEP 2. HOW TO USE POSITIVE STATEMENTS WHEN YOUR CHILD OBEYS:**

Use your positive statements when your child obeys or follows your instructions. Look for opportunities to praise. When you give a command or instruction, give your child immediate feedback and positive remarks as soon as he completes the task. Keep in mind to give only one command at a time. During the time the child is doing the task, do not distract him with questions. A few minutes after the task is completed, repeat the praise. "I will have to tell your father how fast and orderly you returned your games to the shelf." "You were such a big help today." "Your room looks great. I want your grandmother to see this."

Each day create simple, age-appropriate tasks for your child to complete. "Bring me the newspaper from the living room." "Put your backpack in the closet."

These simple exercises give you the opportunity to praise your child and teach him to follow orders. Your positive statements may include: "It's so great to have so much help around the house." "Wow, you did that so quickly." "I am so proud of you. That was great."

This builds a positive self- image and associates happy feelings with following orders. The more praise your child receives, the better chance he will have to learn to follow your instructions and those of other adults.

▶ **STEP 3. HOW TO GIVE EFFECTIVE INSTRUCTIONS:**

Learn to give effective commands. To improve compliance, commands should be simple, short, clear and presented as fact. Do not command in a question form. "Why don't you clean your room now?" should be "Clean your room now."

Only one command at a time should be given to the child. All comments need to be stated in a firm voice and with a matter-of-fact attitude. Neither demand nor threat need be implied in your tone. Make sure each command is fully understood and makes sense to your child. Sometime asking the child to repeat the command will be a way to determine if he understands your instruction.

▶ **STEP 4. HOW TO TEACH YOUR CHILD NOT TO INTERRUPT:**

Teach your child not to interrupt you when you are busy. "I need to talk on the phone. You play alone until I'm finished. Do not interrupt me." A few minutes later, go to your child and praise him for following instructions and being patient. Repeat the same action several times for 10 minutes each time. The next day, repeat same instructions and slowly increase the length of time that he must wait for you to 15–20 minutes. Encourage him to keep busy with interesting activities while he's waiting, and always remember to praise him for waiting so nicely. When he is able to tolerate this for 15–20 minutes without interrupting, you and he are ready for step 5. Even if you are not completely satisfied with his compliance, it's worthwhile to incorporate step 5.

▶ **STEP 5. HOW TO ORGANIZE A HOME TOKEN SYSTEM (REWARD SYSTEM):**

Though many children will respond well to praise and positive feedback, there is a significantly large group that will not respond to praise alone. To improve compliance, a token system is an added incentive. Explain to your child that he is big enough now to get paid for good behavior and tasks that he completes. You are setting up a program in which he can earn privileges/allowance/

treats by completing tasks every week. Compile a list of privileges that will be 'paid' with poker chips. Make a list of age appropriate chores such as setting the table, cleaning his room, getting dressed quickly, coming when called, etc. Now decide how much each chore is worth in chips. A good plan uses about two-thirds of the chips on common privileges and one-third of the chips for a special reward. There should be an opportunity to earn bonus chips for good attitude and really good behavior. Chips will be given only for jobs done on first request and that should be clear to the child. Reward the child for any good behavior, even if it's not on the list, i.e. going to bed cooperatively.

Set up a notebook with seven columns for each day. List the jobs in order, from simple to more complicated, from more frequent to less frequent. As soon as a job is done, add the agreed number of points as soon as possible after completion of the task and add chips to a stack that he can see. At the end of the day, review the total number of points accumulated during the day while reviewing all the tasks that were completed. A big hug and lots of praise should be given when the final results are reviewed.

► WHEN CAN I EXPECT A POSITIVE CHANGE IN BEHAVIOR?

Keep in mind that it's normal to take two steps forward and one back with all children so be prepared for this. This system needs to be operative for at least 3 months before consistent results can be expected. Don't give up. This system brings order, efficiency, responsibility and planning to the life of the child.

Another important benefit to this system is the fact that it can improve the parent-child relationship and help him realize that you are all on the same team. However, if there are siblings, you may need to develop a similar age appropriate program for them, gradually adding more demanding tasks.

▶ WHAT ARE SOME OF THE BENEFITS OF IMPLEMENTING A REWARD SYSTEM?

Although most parents use the program to help manage misbehavior constructively, I feel it is also extremely beneficial to help with organizing and structuring time as well as improving concentration and focus. This system was designed to help instill discipline in a child who seems defiant and refuses to obey parents or teacher. At an early age, we need to understand that children with ADHD are not going to do well with tasks that are lengthy, boring or tedious. The child will lose concentration and fail to complete the task for physiological reasons.

A child does not understand the cause of his limitations and failure which begins the cycle of defiance and frustration, poor self esteem and a lack of confidence. By using this system, defiant behavior can be greatly reduced. This system has an impact on the parents as well. The way a parent responds to defiant behavior can determine the severity of the child's behavior and whether or not there can be a productive outcome.

▶ HOW TO USE THE SYSTEM FOR DISCIPLINE:

To use this system as a form of discipline, the parent should inform the child that when he fails to complete a task expected of him, points or chips will be subtracted. For example: "If you do not begin your homework/clean your room/stop fighting with your sister, by the time I count to three, you will lose points." If the child does not comply immediately, inform him that points/chips are being removed from those he's already earned.

▶ HOW TO USE "TIME-OUT" EFFECTIVELY:

As part of the effort to manage misbehavior, parents can use "time out." More serious misbehavior that has not responded to the point system, use of time out may be effective for children aged 4 to 7. The child should be removed to an isolated location to serve a penalty period. The bedroom or bed should not be used to avoid any negative association with bed time. The use of time-out in the first few weeks needs to be restricted to only one or two forms of misbehavior that did not respond well to other forms of discipline. Focus on changing this particular misbehavior for the next two weeks. You need to count clearly and firmly to 3 after giving the command, stating in a firm authoritative voice that, "if you do not follow my instructions, you will be put in the time-out chair." You must take the child immediately to the 'time-out' chair or a non-stimulating room if these very clear orders are ignored.

During this time he should not be permitted to leave to get a drink, go to the bathroom or use any other stalling tactics. For each year of age, you can apply one minute of time-out time for mild misbehavior and two minutes for serious misbehavior. Do not talk to the child until he is quiet, even if it is longer than one hour. You must not be influenced by tantrums. Once the child has been quiet for a minute past the minimum amount of time in the time-out chair, return to the child with your request. If the misbehavior did not involve a task, but rather an action such as a tantrum or fighting, he should apologize and say he will try not to do it again. Most children will comply. If the child leaves the time-out chair early, return him to it and remain there with him if necessary. This should be followed by a hug and reassurances that you love him very much, but didn't like his behavior. This can be followed by approval for finishing the assigned task. For the rest of the evening, be as positive with your child as possible.

All children become upset with time-out. Gradually they will respond to warnings and the use of time out will decrease. Consistent implementation is the key.

▶ WHAT ARE THE THREE GOLDEN STEPS TO IMPROVE BEHAVIOR?

Children of all ages with ADHD will need help with organizing and planning their day and activities. These golden steps of implementation can go a long way toward improving behavior, reducing frustration and increasing self-confidence.

(1) Defining a Schedule (2) Setting Home Rules (3) Being Organized

▶ **WHAT IS A REASONABLE SCHEDULE FOR AN ADHD CHILD?**

Each child must have a clearly defined schedule. The coaching parent needs to sit and discuss the daily schedule with his child before it is finalized. Have the same routine every day. Let the child know about a change in the schedule as soon as possible to minimize conflict and give the child a feeling of control. "Instead of going straight home after school, we have to go to the doctor/grocery store/etc. first." The parent should sit and discuss the daily schedule with the child before it is finalized. Include homework, play time, outdoor activity, and indoor activity. Post the schedule on the refrigerator door and the child's bedroom and bathroom. It is a wonderful opportunity when reviewing the schedule two or three times a week to develop special quality time with your child. This is a perfect time before bedtime to review some of the activities that he did well and provide positive statements and praise to your child.

▶ **HELP ORGANIZE YOUR CHILD:**

Put your child's frequently used items in order. Have a place for everything and gently insist that he keep everything in its place. When he's finished playing with a toy, have him put it back before getting another. This includes clothing, backpacks, school supplies, toys, sports items, homework and notebooks.

▶ **LEARN TO SET HOUSE RULES:**

Children with ADHD need consistent rules that they can understand and follow. The rules need to be short, simple and clear. When rules are followed, give small rewards. The above three golden steps are essential in helping ADHD children get on equal footing with their peers. A child of four and above can have and should have household responsibilities. Over time, they will be able to take more and more responsibility and you will have less.

▶ HOW CAN I MODIFY CHRONIC POINTS OF CONFLICT?

Children with ADHD have symptoms across a spectrum – from mild to severe. They can be predominantly hyperactive or predominantly inattentive, but all show poor concentration.

A very important behavior pattern for parents to be aware of is that most of these children have a hard time with shifts in activities. This is a major stress. For example, when a child comes home from school and a parent insists that they sit down and do homework immediately, the reaction tends to be very negative. An ADHD child needs time to gradually change from one activity to another. In other words, it is often more productive to say to your child, go play in the yard/watch TV/etc. and I will call you after an hour to start your homework. Even then, you need to give additional notice to the child and let him know that in 15 minutes or as soon as the present TV program is over, it will be time to do homework.

Be aware how easily these children are distracted by any interference or outside stimuli. Providing a serene environment for important tasks such as homework is essential. Special care is needed for any activity associated with risk or danger. Other patterns such as difficulty in following instructions, constantly losing belongings, or appearing not to be listening, seem to be less problematic, but are part of the overall basket of symptoms. Of course, all children lose things or do not always follow instructions, so we are speaking in relative terms.

▶ IMPORTANT POINTS TO REMEMBER:

Praise is the most powerful esteem builder that you have available at a moment's notice.

- Time-out techniques are effective in managing misbehavior and influencing productive behavior changes.
- The three golden steps to improve both behavior and functioning are schedules, organization and clear rules.
- Prepare the ADHD child for transition from one activity to another.

Chapter 12

ADHD AND ASSOCIATED CONDITIONS

Research has shown that up to 50% of parents with preschool age children complain about their children having problems with inattention and hyperactivity. By the time these children reach first grade, the symptoms of inattention and hyperactivity often decrease to a level that is no longer considered as problematic by the parents. About 10% of children who enter first grade continue to show symptoms of ADHD. The majority of those who continue to demonstrate these early symptoms at the age of 6 and 7 will continue to have ADHD symptoms through their childhood and teenage years. The severity of these early symptoms may determine which children will be more likely to show a chronic course of ADHD for the rest of their lives. In the preschool years, most symptoms are confined to inattention, hyperactivity, restlessness, and an excessive need for attention. These children require closer supervision to protect them from possible dangers or accidents. Some of these children demonstrate a high degree of frustration when facing challenges and are often moody and quickly express anger and oppositional behavior. Teachers in daycare often complain of disruptive behavior and difficulty in managing the child.

Entering grammar school places new stresses on a child. These new demands and higher expectations push even children with milder, previously undetected cases of ADHD to their limit, at which point they begin to show clear ADHD symptoms. New demands include sitting still, listening, following instructions, controlling impulsivity and being organized. Often parents are informed by teachers that their child might have ADHD because certain expectations only arise once they are in school.

Many of the academic requirements and some of the social demands of a school setting are above the ADHD child's capacity to manage. The sooner parents are able to provide assistance, understanding and effective treatment, the sooner the child will be able to function effectively in school, reduce social conflicts and minimize any negative impact on self-esteem and personality.

As a child enters school, in addition to, he needs to plan for the next day and take steps to organize his school material, get dressed on time in the morning, etc. Each time a demand is placed on the child that he cannot meet, he will become frustrated and may act out. Simple requirements such as getting dressed, bathing, or preparing to go to school will consume much more time and be more stressful for an ADHD child. Without developed social skills, these children will also suffer rejection classmates and low self-esteem. However, not all children with ADHD show low self-esteem. Some even try to develop an image of unrealistic abilities and even brag about them in an effort to disguise their weaknesses. A very small group of ADHD children will actually show strong and positive self-esteem based on real accomplishment and talent. These children, despite their limitations, are able to function well and to compensate for their deficiencies and succeed. The goal of this book is to increase the number of ADHD children, with or without the additional challenges such as learning disabilities, in this successful group. Parents can look forward to a bright future for their child with effective intervention. The impact of parents on their children cannot be overestimated. Needless to say, the sooner corrective steps are taken, the easier it will be to reach your goals.

Among grammar school students, we are able to identify three groups of children in the spectrum of ADHD. Dr. Beiderman in 1999 found that about 27% of children demonstrate symptoms only to inattention, 7% demonstrate hyperactivity and impulsivity and 59% show both types of symptoms. All the symptoms are not displayed in the same way by all kids but they all have problems with weak neural conduction of stimulatory and inhibitory impulses.

What about the use of medication?

Although medication is effective in reducing symptoms, by itself it does not solve the problem. New research reveals that by the end of the first year, 80% of children are no longer taking any medication. It's true that in about 25% of cases, there is little impact from medication. There is much speculation about the reason and the answer is inconclusive. However, a common reason for medication failure was simply an inadequate dosage or fears about using daily medication in a young child. The strategies discussed in this book make permanent changes in brain function; Ritalin does not. There is no medication for learning disabilities such as dyslexia.

The behavior modification implemented by families seems to have some success in children between the ages of 5–10 years old. Here again, we see that once the program of behavior modification ends, the old behavior returns. Also the child does not carry the new behavior to different but similar situations.

Behavior modification is of limited use unless combined with developing thinking skills, impulse control, memory and concentration. Sessions with therapists are helpful but since the visits are few, the impact on the symptoms can be limited.

Psychotherapy can help adolescents and adults to understand the etiology of their difficulties and may help them find the best solutions and to implement the change. The process is usually quite long and requires the guidance of a therapist throughout. Psychotherapy may not be as effective for young children unless there is depression or anxiety as associated conditions.

The most effective approach is to combine all relevant treatment modalities and to empower parents to take charge of their child's condition and coach him in the skills that are lagging or underdeveloped. The message here is to give parents the skills to take charge, be proactive and coach their child. The heart of this method is to use natural brain exercises to train the child in new thinking strategies, reduce the high level of frustration and increase thinking flexibility, concentration and self control. The fact is, these vigorous exercises would be good for anyone but in a person with ADHD, they are critical.

Once permanent neurological changes occur, the symptoms are alleviated and a remarkable difference occurs in the child's academic performance as well as behavior at home and school. These mental exercises will in no way affect creativity, innovative thinking or any other quality you find so special in your child. In fact, because he will be able to use his time more effectively, develop more social skills and enhance his thinking skills, it's hard to imagine that this will not allow him to devote more energy to developing his innate abilities and talents.

Parents can be the most effective in helping their child and coaching him to overcome the symptoms of ADHD. Any parent can learn the techniques and modify this new approach to fit their child's specific interests, abilities and talents. Proven methods developed at Harvard Medical School and teaching institutions such as the Arrowsmith School as well as others are integrated into a comprehensive treatment for ADHD that makes fun activities for the ADHD child into stimulation for enhancing thinking skills. The use of every day conversations and even crises can be used to re-train or "re-wire" the brain.

Major improvements in treatment and very effective results since 2004 have completely changed our understanding of ADHD. These techniques are the most important development since the use of Ritalin demonstrated that ADHD symptoms could be greatly diminished.

▶ **CONDITIONS ASSOCIATED WITH ADHD:**

If your child also has an associated learning difficulty as well as ADHD, the exercises for ADHD will not impede therapeutic intervention designed for conditions discussed below and in many cases will be complimentary.

The diagnosis and treatment of ADHD is more complicated because the majority of these children have additional associated behavior problems. The prevalence of related or associated symptoms in ADHD children are as follows:

Learning disability	26%
Anxiety disorders	28%
Depression	25%
Oppositional defiance	55%
Conduct disorder	18%

Even though some of the techniques for treating ADHD are extremely helpful to all brain development, each must also have specific remedial efforts to target these complex disorders.

▶ **LEARNING DISORDERS AND ADHD:**

One of the most painful conditions associated with ADHD is learning disabilities. When a child's performance in specific areas such as reading, spelling or math, is significantly below his chronological and mental age level, a learning disability should be investigated. Needless to say, having both a learning disability and ADHD makes schoolwork very challenging. Most ADHD symptoms make studying problematic because of poor concentration, planning and organization. These children cannot be as successful as the other children under these circumstances without intervention. Adding a learning disability to ADHD results in chronic frustration, anger or depression because school work and home work are overwhelming.

There are about three times as many children with ADHD that suffer from learning disabilities as children without ADHD. Like ADHD, symptoms of learning disabilities occur along a continuum, from very mild to severe and come in many different forms. For example, dyslexia is not simply a lag in development that children will outgrow. This condition is an enduring deficit that remains with the child. Since dyslexia is chronic, it is extremely important to identify it early so that a special training program can be implemented. Dyslexia is due to a lack of full development of a specific section of the brain and does not respond to medication. It does not have the same etiology has ADHD nor is it in the same location in the brain. Even though many types of brain stimulation help both conditions, it is very important to intervene with therapy designed specifically for dyslexia or any other type of learning disability.

How can a teacher help?
Avigail Gimpel, M.S.

What is the role of a teacher? This was the question that I grappled with as I entered the noble field more then a decade ago. The choice to become a special education teacher happened quite by accident. I took my first teaching job as a wide eyed enthusiastic and idealistic 20 year old. I was sure I had seen it all and was ready to conquer all challenges. Little did I know what awaited me.

The class was an ESL (English as a Second Language) first grade. The students' ages ranged from six to ten, and most did not share a common language with their fellow students. I had prepared a lovely project for the first lesson, and proudly distributed all of the materials. To my shock and horror, one little boy with wild brown eyes came up right behind me, gathered all the papers, crumpled them up, and threw them out the window. I ignored the outburst, redistributed paper, and began to explain want to do. I had to illustrate the directions on the board due to the lack of common language. A quiet little girl in the corner was completely lost after the first step, and opted to use the Elmer's glue instead to polish her finger nails. She busied herself with that until the end of the lesson. Each time I tried to invite her to join the activity she would do so for a minute, only to get lost again in her glue manicure soon after. A blond boy dropped his scissors which were promptly snatched up by the kid sitting next to him. Without missing a beat, the blond boy jumped on his desk and began kicking the thief in the face. I tried to intervene by grabbing the kid on the desk, and landed up with the pocket of his threadbare shirt in my hand. Things were going from bad to worse.

It was becoming clear that this was not an ordinary class of new arrivals who only needed to learn English. I had stumbled upon a class of students who had a wide range of educational and emotional disabilities. Although my students brought me very close to tears most days, I began growing fond of them. We had been brought together for a reason, and I felt that it was my responsibility not to give up on them. Was I facing the impossible? Was I setting myself up for failure thinking that I could address the diverse assortment of my students'needs. The school guidance counselor tried to encourage me to set up a behavior method of discipline with reward and punishment. I tried giving out candy for good behavior, but besides for the fact that the students usually stole the candy before I got a chance to distribute it, this technique did not sit right with me. Was my goal to teach my students to be quiet so they could get a candy? It did not seem to tackle the real issue -that there was something blocking these kids from behaving or learning. I needed help fast, so I applied to graduate school in Special Education.

My salvation came by way of a visiting professor from Bar Ilan University named Prof. Yaakov Rand. He introduced a ground breaking and novel approach to education that appealed to me right away. His philosophy was based on the work of his brother-in-law, Prof. Reuven Feuerstein, who has been developing his educational approach for over 50 years. Dr. Rand instructed us not to teach, but to mediate. My role as a teacher was expanded from not only imparting knowledge to my students but also explaining the general meaning of the world to the children. I was to guide and help the children understand that the universe has a predictable structure, and understanding that structure would help them navigate through a wide variety of situations in the future.

Every person is modifiable. Throughout life we all develop cognitive functions, or thinking tools, to help us function properly within our environment. We take for granted that we connect events or experiences to each other. If we lacked this skill, each time we had an experience it would be totally new and shocking. Imagine a world so unpredictable and frightening. We naturally develop rules to organize our universe and search for patterns to avoid this sense of chaos. Prof. Feuerstein pinpointed the cognitive functions required for optimal performance and postulated that all learning disabilities stem from deficient thinking skills. This means that all people, no matter what their learning difficulties are, can be taught to overcome them through cognitive exercises.

The first and most vital step on the road to overcome any disability is setting up the proper environment. Feuerstein introduced a system called the Mediated Learning Experience (MLE). The participants in this experience are the child and his caretaker. This could be a parent, grandparent, teacher, baby sitter or even an older sibling.

MLE is a way to enhance and intensify your communication

with your child in a cognitively significant way. Through this method, the caretaker imposes herself between a child and his environment and teaches him how to interpret stimuli in a meaningful way. She also helps a child to express himself, communicate more effectively and become a genuine problem solver. As you embark on this path of enrichment, you will find it not only deeply satisfying, but a lot of fun. Children love to be challenged, and the more you teach them to communicate in a cognitively aware way, the more they and you will benefit from each new experience. You will be helping your child bring order to his inner chaos and solve his learning challenges.

Before we discuss cognitive functions or the actual intervention of MLE, let me illustrate the general learning process. Most of us learn from direct exposure to stimuli. We may also learn from books, friends or teachers, but once we are exposed to new ideas we are able to utilize them freely. If we see a speeding car, we keep out of the way. If we trip on something once, we avoid it the next time. If we speak to someone in a way that gets a bad reaction from him, we try to modify our behavior in future interactions. We learn to read and write through observing and copying letters, comparing them, analyzing their shape, learning the rules and practicing. A human being has a natural need to organize his surroundings, connect events, establish rules and remember past experiences so they can be applied to the future and generally orient himself in space and time. We need these skills to function properly, solve problems, interact with others and have a meaningful existence.

A child with learning disablilties is unable to benefit from direct exposure to stimuli. A caretaker may find himself saying with deep frustration "I have told you this ten times already. Why can't you remember it?" or, "He has seen this letter and learned it just like the rest of his class, yet he continues to invert it." Although it seems as if the child is not listening or can't remember, it may be that this information has not yet become a part of his permanent cognitive structure. He simply cannot receive or retain the information presented because he lacks the cognitive tools to do so. The behavior we are seeing in a child with ADHD is not just a behavior. It is a complex process of impaired cognitive functions that begins when the child is only beginning to tackle any issue. If we treat the behavior (perhaps with a candy or a trip to the Principals office) we have not dealt with the root of the issue, and have only taken a giant step backward in intervention. We do not expect the dentist to fix our teeth without any of his tools, yet we are demanding of a child to perform complex mental processes without teaching him the necessary missing thinking skills needed to accomplish this feat.

To illustrate this point, it often happens that when we learn a new word, suddenly wherever we turn, we hear this word. Did people find out that we learned a new word, and are just helping us along? I doubt it. Although we had heard this word many times before, we did not yet possess the proper tool to connect it to our permanent cognitive structure. Now that we have become aware of it, a new channel has opened, and we are ready to receive it. The same is true for learning a new language. Even those of us who do not suffer from learning disabilities have trouble learning a new language quickly. We first have to lay the groundwork, or structure, for that language by understanding the grammar and rules of that particular language, and only then are we able to build the vocabulary upon it. This is what a baby is doing when he learns his native language. As he learns, he is also establishing the framework and rules for language acquisition. I had this experience when I move to Russia for a few years, and felt like a child with severe learning disabilities. Whereas I had been an effective communicator up until that point, I could no longer open my mouth to say anything useful. Suddenly all the simple functions of life, like shopping or talking on the phone were closed off to me. Direct exposure to the language and culture was of no use to me until I created a mental structure for Russian, (through the assistance of a wonderful tutor) and only then was I able to slowly attach and group words to make sense of them. Interestingly, I was able to learn to read quite quickly despite the different alphabet. This is easily understood because I already possessed the cognitive skills required to read, so I was able to easily apply these same skills of reading acquisition to another language. Once we have mastered a cognitive skill it is easily transferable to different circumstances. This is why cognitive skill acquisition is so vital to effective functioning in life. It was the most shocking experience for a special education teacher to be put in the shoes of my students and understand how the world and its multiple new experiences is closed off to them until we interpret it.

If we pause to analyze the act of thinking, we can see that it takes place in three phases. The first phase is called Input. This is how we gather information, and what we choose to gather. Some obstacles, or deficient cognitive functions, to gathering information are impulsive behavior, lack of need for precision and accuracy in data gathering, and impaired conservation of size, shape, quantity or orientation (direction it is facing). If a child has not gathered complete information, or has gathered it out of order, or can't quite recall its direction or size, it would cause great difficulty in the next phase,

Elaboration is what we do with the data. In most computers, if information is entered incorrectly or too much at once the computer refuses to recognize it. This is called narrowness of the psychic field, shutting down when there is too much information. This is one possibility of a deficient function in the elaboration phase, or unlike a computer a child may continue the thinking process with faulty or incomplete information. He may not be able to define the actual problem, or select relevant cues in defining it. He may have impaired need for pursuing logical evidence so his conclusion would not be based on actual proofs or data provided. These are only a few of the possible impairments that can cause great challenges in thinking.

The final phase is Output, or communication of the best solution. A major cognitive deficiency in communication is an egocentric perspective, meaning that the child only takes his own point of view when communicating. He may offer trial and error responses, or he may be impulsive and act out in response to the problem presented.

These are a few examples of deficient cognitive functions. Keep in mind that a child may have a deficiency in one or more areas. He may have gathered and thought about the data or problem appropriately, but have trouble communicating or vice versa. Once you have identified where the deficiencies lie, and what they are, you are ready for intervention.

As was stated above, MLE is a special way of communicating with a child which enhances his cognitive functions. It has very important criteria, which must be followed in order for the experience to actually correct deficient cognitive functions.

The first step is *Intentionality and Reciprocity*. A parent must intend to engage a child in this cognitive experience, and the child must be aware of it and reciprocate. The parent invites her child to engage in communication on a specific topic.

The second criteria is *Transcendence*. The communication must *not* remain on the level of the actual topic being discussed, but *connect to other areas*. This may be other experiences from the child's own life experience, or other topics with which he is familiar. For example, when discussing problem solving as related to mathematics, the child may bring an example of that same experience of problem solving in the context of sibling rivalry. The steps of identifying the problem, i.e. examining options, choosing the correct solution and checking the results, are the same.

The third criteria is *Meaning*. The topic must have meaning to the child in order for him to retain it. This is how we connect the new information and cognitive tools used to acquire that information to the child's permanent mental structure. If I have connected the seasons with the holidays and the weather we can expect during each holiday, it will become meaningful when the child's birthday is added to that context and placed in context with a holiday and season. Another aspect of creating meaning is to connect the new information to a more general rule, thus imparting to the child a sense of order and the ability assimilate information more effectively in the future.

Below is an example of a real life dialogue of a Mediated exchange between a mother and her children.

Child 1: Mom, what are those things I see at the side of the road that shine?

Mother: those are called reflectors. Do you know what reflectors are? (Here is the mother's *intent* to transmit understanding, and her invitation for the child to *reciprocate*.)

Child 1: no

Mother: A reflector is something that has no light of its own, but shines the light of other lights. Can you think of other reflectors? (The mother is guiding the children to the second stage of *transcendence*, bringing examples of reflectors from other areas.)

Child 2: The moon is a reflector.

Mother: That's right! The moon reflects the light of the sun. Very good example! Can you think of more? (Mother is providing a feeling of competence in child. A note about providing a feeling of competence: it is very good to let a child know what it is you are complimenting him for; not just saying good boy, or you are so smart. If he knows what he has done well he can reproduce it again later. Children also believe compliments when they understand what it is they received it for. The mother also repeats the words of the child so he can hear and reflect upon what he has just said.)

Child 1: At the back of a bicycle there are reflectors.

Mother: Great example of a reflector. Remember when you had to use the bathroom when we were driving at night. Before we got out of the car, what did I put on? (Often we have to assist a child who is struggling to come up with examples. Do not give him the answer, guide him!)

Child 2: That yellow jacket.

Mother: Why do we use it? (intentionality and reciprocity)

Child 2: So people can see us in the dark, because it has reflectors.

Mother: So why do we use reflectors? (This is the very important step which makes it *meaningful* to the child.)

Child 1: So we can be seen in the dark. We don't want people to crash into us or go off the road. Even the moon shows us the way in the dark.

Mother: So we use reflectors to protect us in the dark! (Mother should invite the child to make a rule about reflectors.)

This dialogue is a mediation experience because the child not only received new information, he connected it to the branch of his mental structure about night and protection, he learned to see that the moon and the little reflector on a bike are connected, and see that there is a unity to objects and experiences.

This interaction was initiated by the child, which if you pay attention to your child's questions, it happens very often. But many times the interaction is initiated by the parent.

Examples of entry points into interactions that are child initiated:

1. Child: I want a banana.

   Parent: I notice that you prefer bananas to apples. Why do you think that is? (Intentionality and reciprocity) you may continue by comparing the two fruits, and bringing in other fruit (transcendence) and talk about the nutritional value of each. (Meaning)

2. Child: My brother yelled at me.

   Parent: Why do you think he yelled at you? (Intentionality and reciprocity)

This interaction can go in many directions. It may be positive to try to explore with the child other times this particular brother yelled, what made him behave that way (transcendence- other occasions, and other people behaving in a similar way) and ways of avoiding this experience in the future. (Meaning)

Examples of parent initiated mediation:

Parent: Do you see that traffic light? Do you know what it is for? (intentionality and reciprocity) this can continue by discussing what each color means, and expanded into how the road is organized, bringing examples of other street signs and lines panted on the road (transcendence) and helping the child discover the rules he follows in his every day life (meaning).

Parent to her child when they are baking a cake together: Do you see how the oil spreads when it is poured into the bowl? What other ingredients do the same thing when we pour them into the bowl? How about the flour, does it do the same thing? (Intentionality and reciprocity) This interaction can continue with a discussion of solid, liquid and gas, what they are used for, in a house, in a car, in our own body etc.

What differentiates a mediation interaction from an ordinary conversation? Not all discussions between parents and children can be considered mediation. If a child asks what a reflector is and you define it, you have *not* created a learning experience, and no cognitive functions have been developed or strengthened. Keep in mind that the best way to mediate to your child is through questions. Try to use questions other than "what?" This elicits the more simple cognitive functions, whereas questions such as how, why, how much or when allow you to advance the mediation greatly. Connecting past to present and future is also a valuable way of mediating (remember when…, or what do you think will happen…)

Play time is the most opportune and conducive time for MLE. Play time should not be looked at as a time when the children are out of your hair and you have a few minutes to yourself. A child with learning disabilities had trouble with learning from direct stimuli, so even if you set him up with the most educational video game, the best and the newest in toy technology, chances are he will not benefit very much from the experience. If we as parents are trying to strengthen deficient cognitive functions, play time is the setting that gives us the most opportunities and props with which to accomplish this goal.

A few examples:

1. Organizing Lego into shapes and colors (what is your favorite color, why, what colors do we see most in spring, fall…, can you make a pattern, where do we see patterns, what does this color remind you of…)

2. Playing house (problem solving, imagining scenarios from past, present, future, dressing up and figuring out what clothes are appropriate for different occasions, weather…)

3. Making pictures (learning directions, blending colors, making accurate representations of real life items and events.)

This system is conducive to children with any learning disability because it strengthens the underlying *cause* of the disability, which is the lack of cognitive tools. By practicing this method you will find that not only will your child begin to behave in a more methodical, less impulsive manner, but his other disabilities will begin to improve as well. For more rigorous intervention that directly strengthens each cognitive deficiency there is a system also created by Prof. Feuerstein called Instrumental Enrichment. This involves fourteen instruments including paper, pencil and workbooks that target and exercise deficient cognitive functions. I have worked with students with ADHD and a wide variety of other difficulties with great success using the method of Instrumental Enrichment.

Children love these interactions because they learn in such a natural, unthreatening and positive way. They begin to initiate and request it themselves so it's easy to encourage them to solve problems with siblings and friends using the same interactions. The most wonderful part is that it's simple to do and you will love the interactions and the results.

Many of the treatment strategies of mediated learning experience and collaborative problem solving overlap. Both develop more sophisticated thinking skills and promote brain development, both can be implemented by parents and teachers and both have shown remarkable results. The roots of MLE are in the arena of teaching while the source of CPS and BET are from neurophysiology. They approach developing thinking skills from different vantage points and offer the child both at home and school an optimal learning experience.

► **ANXIETY DISORDER:**

Although anxiety disorders seem to be quite common during childhood when children develop a variety of real and imaginary fears and phobias, for ADHD children, this adds to their difficulties and frustration. Often they are socially awkward and experience rejection by their peer group. The lack of well-developed social skills for their age group, impulsivity and inappropriate behavior clearly demonstrate that these children simply do not know how to play or interact with other children. To avoid these painful encounters, they often avoid school because the experience is riddled with anxiety. The parents and teacher must identify the causes of the anxiety to reduce the pressure on the child and try to teach him to overcome them.

As the child becomes older, the rate of anxiety in general remains the same, but the rate of social phobias can increase. Another developmental disorder that contributes to anxiety is the high level of enuresis (bedwetting) present in ADHD. Usually ADHD children are more dependent on their parents than other children the same age and will show separation anxiety symptoms inappropriate for their age.

The lack of well developed social skills, insecurity and poor self esteem are directly related to constantly struggling and seldom succeeding with the challenges of life. An inordinate level of anxiety may appear right before a task must be performed where the necessary skills are missing or underdeveloped (such as reading in class). These and other facts must be identified and taken into consideration when developing an effective and successful treatment program. The combination of anxiety and unclear thinking is a recipe for explosive behavior, obsessive-compulsive behavior, phobias or rituals that are attempts to reduce anxiety.

► **DEPRESSION:**

Only a few of the children with ADHD show the usual signs of depression. The familiar symptoms of depression like crying spells, sleeping excessively, or being quiet and withdrawn, are not usually seen in these children. Depression is very serious and as many as a third of these children will show signs of depression although it may express itself as high levels of restlessness, anger and agitation. Depression associated with ADHD is more persistent and lasts longer than other types of childhood depression. A 10 year follow up from Harvard University reported in 2005 that children with ADHD have a three to five-fold increase in major depression during their lifetime. Depression that is linked to ADHD has an early onset may persist to adult life. Depression in adult life can obviously be caused by many factors, but it is clearly very prevalent in ADHD children and should be examined in order to initiate early intervention.

► **OPPOSITIONAL DEFIANT DISORDER:**

Inflexibility and poor frustration tolerance look different in different children. The volatility, inflexibility and rigid personality can lead to explosive behavior. Some children deal with stress or developing conflict by leaving the room to avoid acting out or exploding. Numerous 'triggers' may start or cause this oppositional defiant disorder. Difficulty shifting from one activity to another, excessive irritability, certain types of stimulation, discomfort with a new task and frequent conflicts with children in the neighborhood, can easily trigger defiant behavior. The less capable a child is of meeting the demands or requests placed on him, the higher the probability that his reaction will be defiant or immature. Oppositional defiant disorder is more prevalent among boys with ADHD, though many boys without ADHD often show symptoms of this condition at a much lower rate of severity and frequency. These symptoms seem to be the main reason in the U.S. for referral to clinics for evaluation and treatment. Again, all children will express defiance at one time or another; only those whose behavior is so frequent as to seriously impair the quality of life clearly need help.

▶ **CONDUCT DISORDER:**

Without treatment, many ADHD children with oppositional defiance disorder will begin to show signs of conduct disorder with more serious behavioral issues, such as displaced anger directed toward siblings, peers or adults. Sometimes the anger is reflected in cruelty to animals or damage to property. Others will get involved in smoking and drug use while some seek out sexual activity at a very early age. In 2000 a direct link was demonstrated between ADHD children with conduct disorder and close relatives such as mother or father with conduct disorder. These studies and others strongly suggest a genetic component to a child with ADHD and conduct disorder.

▶ **ENURESIS:**

One of the developmental disorders, *enuresis* (bedwetting), seems to be found frequently with ADHD children. Without effective intervention, it is easy to see how this behavior pattern could persist into adulthood, adding to associated conditions like depression or anxiety.

▶ **BIPOLAR DISORDER:**

This is the most serious childhood condition. Children will show signs of irritability, agitation, hyperactivity, anger, highly imaginative and unrealistic thinking as well as heightened aggression and impulsivity. Only 11% of children have been diagnosed as bipolar among those with ADHD. Despite the overlapping symptoms of ADHD and Bipolar in the areas of inattention, hyperactivity and talkativeness, Bipolar disorder and ADHD do not have the same etiology.

▶ **IMPORTANT POINTS TO REMEMBER:**

- When there are one or more co-existing conditions in an ADHD child, treatment is more complicated. However, the treatment strategy must take into account all the behavior issues.
- A small percentage of ADHD children can function well throughout childhood despite their limitations and distinguish themselves later on in life.
- Your child can become a part of this group and you can be the greatest influence toward reaching this goal by implementing and supporting the training and techniques offered in this book.
- Associated conditions will be present in many cases of ADHD and the symptoms associated with it will vary in intensity, frequency and duration just like ADHD symptoms.
- The prevalence of learning disabilities in children with ADHD is about 26%. These two biological conditions exist independently of each other and require two different professional disciplines to handle them effectively.
- Teachers can be the best support for your child.

- Children with ADHD will have three to five-fold risk of developing major depression during their lifetimes.
- Oppositional defiance disorder causes endless stress and conflict for parents and teachers and must be dealt with early and effectively.

Chapter 13

ADOLESCENTS WITH ADHD

You should explain to your adolescent with ADHD exactly what is wrong. If your child had diabetes, you would have to make sure he clearly understood his handicap, how he can help himself and what are the consequences of denial. In many cases where the reason is "hidden" or not discussed, the child assumes he is stupid or slow.

▶ **WHAT ARE THE ISSUES FACING ADOLESCENTS?**

As ADHD has its origins mostly in biology, 70–80% of all children that showed many of its symptoms in grade school will likely continue to display them during adolescence unless there is effective intervention.

All the issues that make adolescence so difficult are that much more complex and challenging for the ADHD child. The rapid physical and hormonal development the adolescent experiences during these years of growth causes constant change in the internal and external image the adolescent is trying to establish. Since the physical changes occur while the emotional development lags, a new source of stress is introduced to the adolescent's life. Developing an identity, yearning for independence, seeking peer group acceptance, dating, school and parental demands are just some of the issues that make the life of most adolescents complicated. For the adolescent with ADHD, this period of life can seem so difficult that many lose direction and even end up in a multitude of crises. This period is by far the most dangerous and stressful time for parents and family.

▶ WHAT ARE SOME OF THE RISKS ADOLESCENTS WITH ADHD FACE?

The combination of poor judgment, impulsive behavior and hyperactivity together with hormonal stress and emotional immaturity create a highly explosive situation for the adolescent with ADHD. Young men with ADHD aged 16–22, have three to four times more traffic citations than the average driver, especially with regard to speeding and crashes. Many of these teens have sexual relations earlier without employing birth control methods, resulting in higher pregnancy rates and sexually transmitted diseases. Because of poor judgment and impulsivity, involvement in risky behavior can even lead to injury or death. The heavy use of cigarettes, drugs and alcohol among this group adds to the degree of difficulties and complexity parents face when dealing with their adolescent child with ADHD.

▶ WHO ARE THE TEENS THAT ARE COMING TO GET HELP?

Teens with ADHD who come to a clinic for help consist of two groups. The first group represents those children that were diagnosed earlier and treated. In other words, they were getting some help in the past and most likely functioned satisfactorily until now. All the changes of adolescence brought increased demands and expectations, resulting in poor school performance, social stresses and misbehavior.

The other group includes all the teens that went undiagnosed until adolescence and coped with ADHD difficulties without getting professional help. As school demands become more complex, the adaptive skills they used during childhood are no longer enough. Depression and anxiety may be ingrained in them quite deeply as they've experienced multiple failures both socially and academically. This can significantly impact character development and increase the risk of developing depression and anxiety later on in life.

▶ CAN ADHD SYMPTOMS BE PRESENTED DURING ADOLESCENCE AS DEPRESSION?

Yes. Most adolescents will be referred for help because of associated conditions that are affecting their interpersonal relationships as well as academic performance.

Lev came to the clinic for evaluation with his mother. She stated that for the past five days he had spent most of his time in bed sleeping and even refused to leave his room to join the family for meals. Fourteen-year-old Lev had clean cut hair and a flat expression on his face. He sat quietly in the office as his mother spoke. Because of her husband's new job in a different city, this was the first year that Lev was attending a new high school. Going to this new school meant Lev had to withdraw from his soccer team and his friends. His grades were satisfactory in his old school, but he did not have any friends in his new school, and reported that he did not like most of his teachers.

His mother noted that he had a very rigid schedule at his previous school. After school, he practiced soccer by himself in the yard for one hour. This was followed by time spent doing homework. Usually it took him much longer to finish his homework than it took his older brother. During this time he would not leave his room, even for meals. He developed his own schedule and kept it rigidly. Any demands placed on him that altered this schedule would cause an emotional outburst. With his father, Lev always had conflicts over changes in his schedule. However, their relationship on the weekends was totally different. Lev's father was a big soccer fan and delighted in seeing how well Lev played. He gave Lev positive re-enforcement and enthusiastically praised him. The mother finished by saying that from the first day in school she noticed that Lev did not have a schedule and became more and more withdrawn. Even his father became concerned and felt that something was wrong and perhaps he was developing some kind of illness. During all this time, while mother was telling the therapist Lev's history, his eyes were fixed on one specific point on the floor. The therapist asked to spend some time with Lev by himself.

Therapist: "You seem to be very sad Lev."

Lev: No response.

Therapist: "Have you ever thought about suicide?"

Lev: For the first time, raises his head from looking at the floor and stared directly at the therapist. "Yes, but I have no plans."

Therapist: "You must feel hopeless to think such thoughts. What bothers you the most?

Lev: "School work always causes me lots of problems. At my old school I put all my effort just to do the work. The new school gave me so much work that I can't do it.

The teachers don't help so much and I have no friends to study with."

Therapist: "It sounds overwhelming."

Lev: "And that's not the worst of it."

Therapist: "Not the worst?"

Lev: "No, soccer was the only things I was good at and I had to give that up."

Therapist: "You must feel like your life is falling apart."

Lev: "That's how I feel."

Therapist: "Have you talked about it with your parents?"

Lev: "Yes, my father told me I played soccer long enough and now it is time to be more serious and get the best education.

We had several fights about it and he always told me that he knew what was best for me."

► **WHAT ARE SOME OF THE FACTORS THAT LEAD ADOLESCENTS WITH ADHD TO DEPRESSION?**

Despite Lev's significant cognitive deficiencies in the area of concentration, he was able to perform adequately although it clearly took him much longer to complete academic tasks. He was able to get by in grammar school and obtained a great deal of positive feedback for his soccer skills. Only when the level of demands placed on Lev outstripped his capacity did he develop depression. The overwhelming loss of positive feedback due to his soccer skills, losing his old friends, heightened academic demands, and poor social and emotional regulation skills all contributed to his depression.

While young children show signs of depression in the form of irritability and agitation, many adolescents begin to exhibit depression with symptoms similar to adults. Poor sleep patterns, loss of appetite, withdrawal, flat affect, feeling down and refusing to communicate are some of the symptoms. Many of the challenges that the adolescent with ADHD faces leave him feeling weak, inadequate and poorly prepared to deal with life's many demands. Poor social and language skills prevent him from dealing effectively with peers. The risk of developing depression for the teen with ADHD is three to five times greater than the general population. Recently I had a boy of 23 referred to me by a colleague for a second opinion whom he had been treating for depression. This boy's history told a sad but familiar story. He's 23 years old, had been kicked out of one of the most prestigious religious schools in Jerusalem. The pieces of his story did not fit: He had grades of 95 in some subjects and failing in others. He spoke about his inability to complete tasks and day dreaming. He was gifted in music and that was his main feeling of accomplishment.

He applied for jobs below his ability level but seldom held a job for more than a few months. Even when he got a position in music school, he was unable to do well. Poor social and family relationships were evident. Further evaluation led to the diagnosis of ADHD with, of course, depression, poor self esteem and all the emotional results of so many years without treatment.

▶ HOW DOES ANXIETY IMPACT ADOLESCENTS WITH ADHD?

Anxiety is another condition frequently seen in adolescents but is more extreme in those with ADHD. Recognizing weaknesses and deficiencies can explain the high rate of this associated condition. Although anxiety symptoms such as fear and stress are not as debilitating as other conditions, their presence reduces the adolescent's overall level of functioning and self-confidence. To reduce the level of anxiety, many adolescents increasingly turn to alcohol and smoking. Anxiety, low self esteem and poor judgment push the adolescent toward risky behavior.

▶ THE IMPACT OF OPPOSITIONAL DEFIANCE DISORDER ON ADOLESCENTS WITH ADHD:

Oppositional Defiance Disorder (ODD) is one of the more problematic conditions associated with ADHD. If not handled correctly, it can lead to conduct disorder and adult anti-social behavior. ODD in the early adolescent years is so prevalent among boys that almost 60% of all teens exhibit many of the symptoms. At the same age, only 35% of girls will exhibit similar symptoms. What makes this condition so problematic is the fact that during these years all adolescents exhibit some degree of oppositional and defiant behavior as part of normal growth and maturation. However, because of poor judgment, emotional immaturity and impulsive behavior in the ADHD teen, the mistakes made can be more serious and the consequences much more severe. Behavior patterns caused by this condition seem to be the most frequent trigger for conflicts between parents and teens.

▶ **IMPACT OF ANTI-SOCIAL BEHAVIOR ON ADOLESCENTS WITH ADHD:**

As untreated adolescents with ADHD grow older and reach young adulthood, more than 30% continue to show dysfunctional behavior and exhibit conduct disorder symptoms. From this group of ADHD adolescents, about 8% of the girls and 20% of the boys show aggressive and destructive episodes. They will be involved in lying, stealing and vandalism. Parents and other authority figures will face conflict and explosive behavior from this group of teens. Dr. Beiderman found that a high percentage of the adolescents that display conduct disorder behavior, were diagnosed with oppositional defiance disorder as young children. The increased family conflict and decreased family cohesion were associated with it as well. Family genetic risk factors may account for the onset of conduct disorder in some cases. This group must receive professional help. Without proper management one can expect constant conflict with parents, school officials and the legal authorities.

▶ **WHY DO ADOLESCENTS WITH ADHD HAVE AN INCREASED RATE OF SMOKING?**

The association of maternal smoking during pregnancy and increased risk factors for ADHD in children was reported for the first time in 1997. Mothers who smoked during pregnancy have a 22% risk of bearing children with ADHD. Mothers who did not smoke have a risk rate of only 8%. The presence of nicotine in the nervous system actually improves concentration. Nicotine stimulates the increased release of brain neurotransmitters resulting in some improvement in concentration, anxiety relief and general nervous feeling. Despite the mild benefit of nicotine on the nervous system, it should be emphasized that smoking causes much more damage than benefit and should be avoided at all costs. Some ADHD children start by age 10 and by the age of 18, more than 50% of ADHD teens will be smoking as compared to 20–23% of adolescents without ADHD. It has been shown that teens who smoke are 12 times more likely to try other drugs. Beiderman demonstrated that treating adolescents with Ritalin continuously for several years reduces the chance that these adolescents will start smoking. At the same time, follow up of a group of adolescents with the same condition who did not receive Ritalin for their condition showed that 13% of the group began smoking. Receiving medication significantly reduced the risk of starting to smoke.

▶ WHY DO ADOLESCENTS WITH ADHD HAVE A HIGHER RATE OF DRUG AND ALCOHOL ABUSE?

As with smoking, the increased rate of substance abuse in ADHD teens is dramatic. By age 15, the rate of alcohol and drug abuse is double the rate of teens without ADHD. This statistical correlation continues to age 20. The high rate of substance abuse by the ADHD adolescent who does not receive any treatment raises the question as to whether drugs are used to self-medicate in an attempt stave off distressing feelings. Nicotine, alcohol and street drugs are known to impact the same area of the brain where the ADHD adolescent has deficiencies. This mild benefit does not justify the serious and often permanent damage to the brain, as well as other organs, caused by heavy drug use. All efforts need to be made by parents to preempt the use of these dangerous chemicals. Do not assume it is a stage that will be outgrown. Far better to use Ritalin and implement BET and CPS as well as the other strategies than to have the child "self-medicate" with alcohol, nicotine and street drugs.

The use of Ritalin does indeed impact the rate of adolescent drug abuse. Studies show that among medicated and treated

ADHD adolescents, alcohol and drug abuse was limited to 10% whereas similar un-medicated adolescents with ADHD showed a shocking rate of 35% (as compared to 8% of adolescents without ADHD). It may be that they are medicating themselves with street drugs to get relief from their symptoms.

▶ HOW DO LEARNING DISABILITIES IMPACT ADOLESCENTS WITH ADHD?

Learning disabilities in the areas of reading, writing, spelling and math can appear separately or together in an ADHD teen. While these associated conditions do not pose a direct risk or danger, they can cause severe frustration and poor self-esteem and limit his potential, which in turn can lead to anxiety, depression and acting out. As many as 30% of males and 12% of females with ADHD will show this associated condition, which only appears in 10% of the general population.

Some parents and teachers confuse these two conditions. Learning disabilities and ADHD are two separate and independent conditions caused by mild brain irregularities in different parts of the brain. The brain center controlling reading skills has been clearly identified and is located in a different area of the brain, quite removed from the ADHD area. A learning disorder can place serious limitations on an adolescent's school performance. While many ADHD children are able to compensate in a variety of ways for their learning disabilities during the grammar school years, at a high school level, it often becomes too difficult. Many of the conflicts in early adolescent years are triggered by academic and school demands. This is why it is so important to treat both conditions at the same time and as early as possible.

Parents need to recognize the academic limitations of an ADHD teen. When the adolescent is confronted with work he can not do successfully, it is less painful to state to parents "I do not want to do this assignment" or "I do not want to go to school," rather than admit, "I can't do the work." Being oppositional and defiant on this subject actually helps him feel more independent. To him, admitting that he cannot do the work would be admitting that he can't keep up with the other kids in his class. It should be emphasized that a learning disability does not mean that a child is stupid; often they have a high IQ. But understanding the disability will allow one to begin to form a working academic plan.

Adolescents with ADHD and a learning disability will have to receive tutoring on an intense regular basis. Up to 95% of the teens in this group will need special academic assistance to graduate high school. Participation in special classes or remedial programs should be done in a matter-of-fact way as part of the school or academic year.

▶ WHY DO ADOLESCENTS WITH ADHD HAVE FOUR TIMES AS MANY CAR ACCIDENTS?

Teenagers, especially boys, begin talking about driving before they even turn 16. Every teenager, including those with ADHD, would like to start driving as soon as possible. Parents need to know that teenagers and young adults with untreated ADHD are at great risk to themselves and others when they are behind the wheel of a car. Noncompliance with the rules of the road, lacking focus, being easily distracted and acting impulsively are clearly hazardous for the driver and the general public. The National Highway Traffic Safety Administration recently reported that automobile accidents are the leading cause of death for teenagers. Motor vehicle accidents account for about 36% of all deaths of people ages 16–20. About 45% of the fatalities occur because of excessive speed. Research found that teenagers with ADHD are nearly *four times* more likely to be involved in a motor vehicle accident. A study by the American Academy of Pediatrics comparing adolescents with and without ADHD show that the ADHD group has more automobile accidents, more bodily injuries, are more often at fault, receive more traffic citations, and are four time more likely to get a speeding ticket.

▶ **HOW TO PROMOTE SAFE DRIVING AMONG ADOLESCENTS WITH ADHD:**

A study conducted by researchers at the Washington Neurological Institute found that adolescents with ADHD who were given long-acting methylphenidate once a day improved their driving safety performance by improving concentration and focus.

Some suggestions for increasing attention and decreasing unsafe driving habits for all adolescents are as follows:

- Keep the cell phone in the trunk of the car while driving.
- Set the radio before starting to drive and do not change the station.
- Avoid peak driving hours
- Plan trips in advance
- Limit passengers in the car to one.

Parents who think they may have an untreated adolescent with ADHD need to have him carefully diagnosed and treated for his own safety and the safety of others.

▶ **WHAT ARE THE THREE TOPICS PARENTS NEED TO UNDERSTAND ABOUT ADOLESCENT ADHD?**

Dealing effectively with the normal challenges of adolescence can be very difficult. These issues will be dramatically magnified when parents are dealing with teenagers with ADHD. Before parents can seek solutions for the conflicts with teenagers, they need to understand three topics:

- Adolescent developmental issues
- ADHD symptoms and their impact
- Their teen's strengths and weaknesses.

▶ **WHAT ARE THE ISSUES FACED BY ALL TEENAGERS?**

- Identity formation and character development
- Socialization skills and friendships
- Setting educational goals
- Coping with strong sexual urges

- Temptations of smoking, drugs and alcohol
- Increased academic demands
- Family relationships
- Learning to become independent and separate from parents.

The above tasks are faced by all adolescents but the ADHD adolescent is less prepared to deal with them because of underdeveloped skills. Because of poor ability to regulate emotions, ADHD adolescents may be extremely volatile and explosive. Although the ADHD adolescent seeks independence, he will not be able to assume the responsibilities that independence requires. He will need guidance and assistance and will likely resent it. His poor organizational and planning skills as well as poor problem solving and forethought will lead to school and family conflicts.

You must keep the above information all the time in your mind so that you can keep your own emotions under control. Most parents become angry, lose control and fuel conflict unnecessarily. If you have a firm understanding of your teen's weaknesses, this will help you adjust to realistic academic expectations and bolster his self-confidence in areas where he can excel.

▶ **LEARN TO RECOGNIZE YOUR ADOLESCENT'S STRENGTHS:**

The most important way to help your teen recognize his capabilities and talents is to assess his strengths and help him to develop them. The key to reducing conflict during the adolescent years is to focus on the positive. If your teen does not naturally gravitate toward an extracurricular activity, help him develop one. If your teen is small, encourage activities like gymnastics and karate rather than football or basketball. You are in a position to observe your child for years and can make note of his strengths. Focus on his strengths and encourage independent activity in any area that provides him with feelings of success and accomplishment. He may not find it by himself.

► **WHAT ARE SOME OF THE COMMON CAUSES OF CONFLICT WITH ADHD ADOLESCENTS?**

Some of the more common foci of conflict are:
- Homework and school related issues
- Socializing with appropriate friends
- Use of nicotine and drugs
- Respect of family members
- House rules, routine and chores
- Curfew time and appropriate behavior

These most likely will be issues in your house. Add to the list any additional topics that precede conflict. Keep in mind that most adolescent ADHD actions are unpredictable and are not done intentionally to upset parents. Teens do things for a variety of reasons. If you interpret their actions as malicious, you will be angry and not effective. Keep your cool.

► **WHAT ARE REASONABLE HOUSE RULES?**

All adolescents need to have structure and boundaries. All adolescents with ADHD will function poorly without them. Rules must to be clear, short and simple. Negotiating rules that everyone can live with seems to be the best way to go. The teen understands the reason for the rules and his part in the well being of the family. You will have your own set of priorities for house rules but the following are good examples.

Examples of House Rules:
- No inappropriate language
- No smoking
- Parents must always know whereabouts and plans
- Come home by curfew time
- Respect parents
- Household responsibilities

Go over the list several times with your teen and discuss the reasons and necessity for each rule. These rules need to be posted in a visible place. One should begin this around age 12. The older the child, the more difficult it is to institute and the more patience will be needed. Both parents must take the same position in enforcing the rules. With many teens, it's helpful to associate this with a regular allowance. You can have a positive discussion by pointing out all the rules he already follows and discuss ways to prevent conflict in the future.

Adolescents needs positive feedback so it's always good to praise him for anything and everything he does for the family and by adhering to the rules and not causing them to worry. Every opportunity that justifies praise, even for small matters, is positive. Try to focus on actions related to independence and responsibilities as well as any action taken that reflects planning and self-control.

▶ **PLAN OF ACTIVITIES AND SCHEDULE FOR THE WEEK:**
One of the most useful tactics to develop together with your teen is a weekly schedule. A major effort needs to be given to outside organized activities. When we study biographies of successful adults with ADHD, we see a common feature. Most of them were very involved with organized activities during adolescence. These activities included participating in youth organizations, sports clubs, dance classes, sport teams.

The feedback and positive re-enforcement they receive help to balance the less than stellar academic performance. The need to identify with a group and to feel a part of it is important during these years. Teenagers need to feel more independent from parents and to form a positive self-image. The main reason parents should provide direction is to prevent a teen from falling in with the wrong group. Unfortunately, because of poor judgment and emotional immaturity, the group may be a marginal one whose identity revolves around undesirable behavior such as drugs, alcohol and/or promiscuous sexual activity.

Since homework is a major cause of stress and conflict, regular daily free time needs to be a part of the regular routine. Computer time is an activity that most ADHD children should include in a daily routine. Computers can be an excellent resource because they are non-judgmental, providing visual stimulation and improving concentration. Since "smart" video games have been shown to increase blood flow and neuronal connection,. learning computer skills can also give an additional positive sense of accomplishment because it is an independent activity and mistakes will not cause the same degree of stress. Use games involving strategy, not violence.

Try to schedule a weekly meeting to review the week and handle past or potential conflicts or challenges. Most adolescents will resist this activity, but try to implement it casually, whenever the opportunity presents itself. Free time in the possession of the ADHD adolescent is often not used productively. Find activities where he can do well, improve his self-esteem and develop organizational skills. There should be limits on the amount and content of TV. A favorite program can be a reward for the completion of homework, chores or other responsibilities.

► **ASSIGNING HOUSEHOLD CHORES:**

Every teen needs to contribute to the family. Chores such as cleaning, taking out the trash, helping younger siblings, setting the table, clearing the table, etc. should be part of a daily routine. This schedule can be presented as a way to create more time for fun activities, with each chore taking no more than a few minutes. This can also be a good opportunity for praise. For example, for younger teens simple household chores can get positive feedback. "You always do a great job of setting the table and I noticed it takes you less than five minutes." Older teens that take care of younger siblings should know that their help is appreciated. The schedule should be a collaborative effort and any complaints negotiated.

► HOW CAN SELF-ESTEEM BE BUILT IN AN ADHD ADOLESCENT?

Genuine self-esteem will come as a teen develops his identity and accomplishes goals. This is a slow, often painful process. Teens are quite dependent, know it and resent this dependence. There will be many attempts to demonstrate his separation by challenging his parents on a regular basis. Most parents become angry and misinterpret this behavior as disrespect. As educated parents, you need to view this as the teen's natural attempt to separate from the family and show external signs of independence even though, of course, it is just a façade. True independence is many years away and can be accomplished if the parents remain calm and in control and help guide their child toward independence. If parents fail to do this, the teen will look for activities that will give him a feeling of independence and belonging. Drugs, alcohol and smoking as well as joining marginal groups that will accept him and re-enforce his need to belong can always be found. As long as parents keep this in mind, a consistent plan of action can be implemented.

The best way to build a positive and strong self-esteem is to accomplish goals. The more goals an adolescent with ADHD, or any adolescent for that matter, can accomplish, the better he will feel about himself. Often the parent, because of wider experience and knowledge, will know many activities that will re-enforce the natural abilities of their child or initiate activities that will allow him to develop specific skills.

Real accomplishments through hard work should always be praised and encouraged. Let him know how proud you are.

With a collaborative effort, realistic and rewarding goals can be set. Most parents try to encourage their children to "do their best." This approach does not help develop positive self-esteem or reduce the level of anxiety and pressure. The instruction "to do your best" is confusing to the ADHD child because he does not know exactly what his best effort is. You are able to set an attainable goal that will contribute to positive self-esteem is by defining the goal specifically. Be sure that the goal is realistic and attainable.

▶ HOW TO DEFINE REALISTIC GOALS:

Parents need to capitalize on the capabilities of their child. Earlier we pointed out the importance of knowing the strengths and weaknesses of each child so that the parents and child can be realistic in their expectations and determine specific goals. If you know your child's ability level, then set the goal at 10% below his best effort. The actual number is not so important; what is important is successful completion of the task with hard work and the feeling of accomplishment. If you find it difficult to ascertain the strengths of your child, consider an aptitude test to clarify his strengths, ask teachers, coaches and other adults that are involved. Find activities after school that gives him the opportunity to strengthen his skills. For an adolescent with ADHD, every success builds self- esteem and compensates for areas where he is weak. Another approach should be to have short -term goals, i.e. to accomplish the designated goal in a week. Do not talk in terms of long -term goals (the end of the year, for example). If the task requires a long period of time, break it into sections. For example, a book report or term paper due by the end of the school year can be divided into an introduction and the first few following chapters. Try to set goals in areas where the teen shows interest and has some motivation. It is much more important to play on strengths. This doesn't mean you allow your child to ignore reading or math just because it is an area where he is weak, but you do need to find areas where he can get positive feedback and experience success. Encourage after school activities such as Scouts or sports.

▶ HOW TO CAPITALIZE ON EVERY ACCOMPLISHMENT:

Many ADHD adolescents make positive contributions both at school and at home. However, it seems to be human nature to immediately react and criticize any misbehavior and forget to praise and appreciate. It's really very difficult to over-appreciate or say too many words of praise for all the small things that are done each day. By recognizing each and every successful effort, you present him with an emotional reward. Each reward one receives causes a real chemical reaction in the brain and re-enforces positive change. Make an objective assessment of how often each day you make positive statements of praise and encouragement, appreciation and support. Invite your child to go jogging with you as well.

▶ THE IMPORTANCE OF OUT-OF-SCHOOL ORGANIZED GROUP ACTIVITIES:

As a parent, your goal is to find as many activities as possible that will build your child's self esteem. Organized activities offer a ready-made system for building physical, mental and social skills.

Activities that involve vigorous physical exercise have countless benefits to ADHD children as well as teenagers and adults. In addition to the benefits that come from having a healthy body, these activities help the ADHD individual to focus, increase neurotransmitters and stimulate neuronal connections in the same areas of the brain where the ADHD child shows deficiencies. You will see that all teenagers have a need to be part of a group of their peers. Without parental guidance and the development of a positive self image, ADHD teenagers are more likely to join marginal groups. Parents are able guide their children into activities that will enhance their lives, develop skills and provide them with a sense of accomplishment and belonging. Needless to say, it is much easier to influence a teenager of 13 than 17. The sooner these habits and activities are in place, the greater their benefit and chance of success.

▶ WHICH GROUP TO JOIN?

Joining any type of sport club will be very productive if it is matched with your teen's strengths. You should try to assess the personality and character of the coach to see that he or she will be a positive influence and role model. Explain the cause and treatment, why the coach's relationship is so important and how to communicate effectively with your child.

Youth movements such as the scouts can potentially be an excellent opportunity to develop social as well as leadership abilities. Joining organizations that specialize in volunteer activities can give the ADHD teen a special sense of worth. Joining any productive organized activity can contribute to an overall improvement in skills, socialization, and sense of belonging. All of these will enhance self-esteem.

▶ **WHAT CAN I DO IF MY CHILD REFUSES TO JOIN ORGANIZED GROUP ACTIVITIES?**

Some teens may refuse to join organized activities. Of course, the younger the child is, the easier it is to influence him. Many children will fear activities with a new group. Several strategies can be developed to overcome their resistance. First, the organized activity needs to match the child's capabilities and interests. If the child has no particular interests, find out what activities his schoolmates or cousins are involved in and see if you can interest him in the same thing. Parents need to nurture any type of minimal interest in activities gradually but persistently.

The next step is to choose activities that are accessible to you and your child. The final step is to contact the group leader for a meeting. A group leader is the key person to successfully integrate your child into the group. He can have a very meaningful influence on your child.

You can also investigate volunteer groups that provide support to children with handicaps in hospitals or day centers. If your child is in his early to mid-teens, this can be a very positive experience at many levels. This can give him a sense of responsibility and satisfaction from helping others less fortunate. Following these strategies may make the entry into new activities smoother.

► **SPECIAL PARENT-TEEN ACTIVITIES:**

Whenever possible, mothers should take daughters and fathers their sons, for special activities they can enjoy together. These activities will strengthen the relationship with the parent, re-enforce the identity of the child and develop a feeling of maturity. Try to pick activities that are associated with maturation. "You are old enough now to take a trip out of town with me/ go with your brother to a movie at night/ take the bus to the park with your friends.

This kind of interaction will give the teen the feeling of being special, improve positive interaction and indicate that he is growing without the need to create conflict.

► **CHANGE YOUR ATTITUDE AND BEHAVIOR:**

A key component to help the ADHD teen develop strong self-esteem is parental interaction. The development of a positive relationship is a must, but how? All children need to feel unconditional love and acceptance. You may not like his behavior, it should never change your unconditional love, and he should know it. You must respect your teen and let him know you want to treat him respectfully, and help him to understand his condition. Be open, honest and optimistic to encourage cooperation. Establish a habit of regularly discussing issues without complaining. Develop positive communication. It is very easy to lose control during a disagreement or conflict. Listen carefully to make sure you fully understand the issues, state your case clearly and briefly and do not criticize. When talking, take turns; have a conversation, don't give a lecture. Keep calm and talk in a normal tone of voice. Don't dredge up the past. Focus on the present.

Following the above recommendation will help your adolescent relate to you in a more productive manner and begin to take steps to compensate for many of his deficiencies. This will help reduce associated conditions like anxiety, depression or conduct disorder.

► **IMPORTANT POINTS TO REMEMBER:**

- Vigorous mental and physical exercises are crucial for teens. Refer to children's section.
- All the issues that make adolescence so difficult for most children are more complex and challenging for the ADHD teen.
- The combination of poor judgment, impulsive behavior and hyperactivity together with hormonal changes and emotional immaturity is an explosive mixture that can lead to chronic conflict and disagreement.
- Most adolescents will be referred for help because of one of its associated conditions that causes problems in the family, social and/or academic areas of their lives.
- As many as 20% of all ADHD adolescents show serious signs of depression during the teen years.
- A high number of adolescents demonstrate oppositional defiant disorder. If not effectively treated, this group will have an increased risk of substance abuse, smoking and anti-social behavior.
- ADHD teens are more than twice as likely to smoke and are 12 times more likely to use drugs and alcohol.
- Medical treatment during adolescence with methylphenidate has been shown to reduce alcohol and drug use by 50% and even prevent smoking.
- Among those with ADHD, the likelihood of associated learning disability is as high as 30%. The presence of this associated condition will make academic work very difficult.
- Adolescents with ADHD who do not receive treatment face a real risks. They are four times more likely to be involved in a fatal accident than an adolescent without ADHD.
- Establishing reasonable house rules is the first step to bringing some degree of stability to the home and reducing conflict and stress.
- Working together with a teen on a weekly schedule will

bring more order and organization into the life of the teen and the family.

- Define and help accomplish realistic goals to build self-esteem.
- All adolescents will benefit from strong affiliation with after-school organized group activities – sports, youth movements, dance, acting, etc.
- Collaborative problem solving is an effective way to handle many of the adolescents with ADHD.
- Think of physical activities you can do with your child or that involve the whole family.

Chapter 14

COLLABORATIVE PROBLEM SOLVING WITH ADOLESCENTS

▶ **COLLABORATIVE PROBLEM SOLVING (CPS) AS A FORM OF TREATMENT:**

As children mature, many of their hyperactivity symptoms diminish. However, impulsivity and inattention persist for ADHD teens. By far the most common problem most parents face with ADHD adolescents is defiance and oppositional behavior. Conflict about school and homework, conflict with parents and siblings and acting out with peers, are common and often major sources of disruption.

Learning to handle oppositional behavior skillfully is a must for parents of ADHD teenagers. It is often a confusing bewildering time for parents who feel they are watching a train wreck in slow motion.

There are some medications that can reduce emotional outbursts. However, no medication can change defiant and hostile behavior toward authority figures. The most effective method to deal with defiant disorder is to use the Collaborative Problem Solving (CPS) approach. This type of behavior has been described by Dr. Ross Greene as a delay in the development of flexibility and frustration tolerance. The lagging development of the prefrontal area of the brain and the deficiency in neurotransmitters delays the full development of age appropriate cognitive skills:

To master these complex skills, one needs to develop or improve his abilities in all five domains. This needs to be practiced over and over consistently just as you would with any other skill.

1. Cognitive Flexibility Skills:
    A range of perception rather than black and white.
    Adapting to change.
    Objectivity in point of view.
    Accepting mistakes as a part of life.
2. Social Skills:
    Reading verbal and nonverbal cues.
    Adapting to group activities.
    Understanding how one's behavior affects others.
    Seeking attention in productive ways.
3. Executive Skills:
    Handling transition from one activity or emotion to another.
    Staying on topic.
    Doing functions in order.
    Sorting through thoughts.
    Learning the consequences of actions.
    Shifting from one mind set to another.
4. Language Processing Skills:
    Verbally expressing emotions, i.e. frustration, anger, sadness, etc.
    Expression of needs and concerns.
    Clear, organized expression of thoughts.
5. Emotional Regulation Skills:
    Management of anxiety, depression.
    Management of moods.
    Limiting emotional reactions to the cause.

Remaining positive in other areas of life when faced with difficulties.

► **TEACH YOUR TEEN TO DEVELOP COGNITIVE SKILLS:**

The lagging development of cognition in ADHD individuals can be overcome with the proper coaching. Just as a teenager works out to develop physical strength, so too can he develop the cognitive skills he needs with coaching from parents. Just as it takes time and persistence to develop physical skills, it takes practice to develop cognitive skills. Regardless of the situation, when cognitive demands on an ADHD teen outstrip his capacity to respond adaptively, he will show explosive behavior.

As his cognitive skills strengthen, the teen will be able to handle more demanding challenges. Behavioral approaches such as reward and punishment will have no real long-term benefit to s teen with cognitive deficits because new skills must be acquired in order to change future behavior. It's important to internalize that the ADHD teen's behavior is not manipulative or attention seeking. By identifying specific cognitive skills that are lagging, one can focus on developing the skills that need to be acquired to prevent maladaptive responses, outbursts and explosive behavior.

► **THE THREE METHODS PARENTS USE TO SOLVE PROBLEMS:**

When facing difficult issues, parents have three options:

Option 1: The controlling parent who believes his children should follow his instructions without question. For the ADHD teen, this approach will lead to poor results. Even though he may respond to this approach and some parental expectations may be met, the price is high in terms of anger, frustration, and emotional outbursts. More important, no new skills are acquired, so when confronted with similar issues in the future, the teen will not be better equipped to solve the problem.

Option 2: The permissive parent may elect to preempt outbursts and conflict passively by dropping demands. An outburst may be avoided this way, but again, no new skills will have been learned.

Option 3: A life skill is developing the ability to find the best solution to problems. We are going to be training and strengthening lagging skills by using the collaborative problem solving (CPS) method. When using all four steps in the proper order, CPS can accomplish three goals:

1. Reduce explosive outbursts
2. Help teen meet adult expectations
3. Develop flexibility, frustration tolerance and other thinking skills that are lagging skills.

When is the best time to start CPS?

Better results with CPS can be achieved when the approach is used in a proactive way. When parents or therapists can correctly identify specific conflicts and wait for a time when both parents and teen are under little stress. This is the best time to introduce the conflict with the intent to understand the problem and find a solution. When both participate equally in the process, finding the best solution can begin without antagonism.

▸ **DEVELOP A UNIFIED POSITION WITH YOUR SPOUSE BEFORE STARTING CPS:**

Before introducing the four steps used to succeed with CPS, a healthy atmosphere must exist in the house. Effective preparation by the parents before coaching their teen is essential. Parents need to agree on the same method of approach, be consistent and establish unity in dealing with the adolescent. Once parents agree to use CPS, they must give up other methods and approaches. You can't use a dictatorial approach one day and the CPS method another.

Approach your teen with both acceptance and a clear

understanding of how and why he is different. Accepting the fact that he has this condition will remove pressure and unrealistic expectations from him and from you. Understanding the etiology of your teen's difficulties means that you are not a poor parent and he is not bad/lazy/uncaring. This is the first and most important step on your road to helping your child.

► **THE FIRST STEP IN THE CPS APPROACH:**

Four steps are involved in this approach to resolve conflict and at the same time develop skills:

Empathy and Reassurance:

Adolescents with ADHD tend to be very sensitive and emotional. Showing empathy to the stressed teen is the first step in establishing positive communication and creating a better atmosphere for productive exchange. Empathy will help the teen remain calm. Statements like, "I'm not going to talk to you until you calm down." or "Go to your room" are not productive and will not create a better atmosphere. Empathy will reassure your teen that you are aware of his stress and intend to listen to him. How can you express empathy? By showing understanding and repeating what he has told you. Below is a description of a possible approach to a crisis:

Teen: "I am not going back to school."
Parent: "You don't want to go back to school."
Teen: "I am not going to clean my room today."
Parent: "You don't want to clean your room today."
Teen: "I am not speaking to Sarah anymore."
Parent: "You are not going to speak to Sarah anymore."
Another approach is to state your observations:
"You're very upset right now."
"You are very angry and frustrated."
"Sarah must have hurt your feelings."
By expressing empathy, you are taking a neutral position that

by itself is very reassuring. You have not taken any position. You are not agreeing or disagreeing with the teen.

Sometimes the adolescent will complain about you. Statements like: "You are ruining my life." "It is all because of you."

You can respond "I hear you." "I seem to cause you a lot of stress."

An adolescent may come with extreme demands or a negative response to your request. Statements like: "I am not going to do…" or "I want to go out with my friends," can be countered with "I am not saying you have to…" or "I am not saying no." This leaves the door open to begin a dialogue. Of course you have not said yes to the demands or acquiesced to the refusals either. You need your teen to be involved if you are going to solve the problem together. Your goal in this first step is to engage your teen in a calm quiet exchange.

► **THE SECOND STEP IN CPS:**
Define the Problem and Articulate Concerns:
Once you have an engaged and willing adolescent, the second step is to understand and define the issue at hand. Most problems can be negotiated and a solution found that can be tolerated by both. To continue in a positive way, the parent must express concern for the teenager and help him think and express his needs. The opening statement can be as simple as "What's going on?" "What is bothering you?" "What's on your mind?"

Some adolescents will be able to express their concerns, but most will need guidance to develop clear thoughts and express what's wrong.

Crisis Resolution:
It's worthwhile considering the following scenario as an example of how a crisis might be resolved.

Adolescent: "I had a bad day at school and I'm not going back."

Parent: (initial empathy) "You are not going back to school?"

Adolescent: "That's right. You can't make me."

Parent: "What is going on at school?"

Adolescent: "I had a big fight with my teacher and he sent me out of the class."

Parent: "Mr. Hellman sent you out of the class."

Adolescent: "Yes, he did. He asked me for my homework and I didn't have it and he sent me out of the class."

Parent: "For not turning in your homework, he sent you out of the class."

Adolescent: "Yes. I got so mad at him that I said I don't care and I cursed."

Parent: "It seems you lost your temper and exploded in class in front of all the students."

Adolescent: Yes, that's why I do not want to go back to school."

Parent: "I understand that you are very embarrassed and do not want to go back to school. I didn't say you have to go back to school, but not going back to school might mean you'll have to repeat the whole year."

Notice that it took several steps for the parent to guide the teen to identify the real problem and define it clearly.

Many adolescents and parents tend to state their solution before working the problem through. For example, the adolescent's decision not to return to school is his solution. A parent must make sure that the real concern is clearly defined and stated. In the beginning a parent will have to take an active role to help his teen define the problem and the consequences of his actions. At this stage, we have two defined opposing concerns openly presented to the adolescent, the adolescent being embarrassed to return and face the class and the parent concerned with the loss of the academic year. The adolescent is focused on the short-term crisis while the parent is focused on long-term consequences.

► **THE THIRD STEP IN CPS:**

Considering a Range of Solutions:

In this step, the teen is invited to suggest possible solutions to the problems and verbalize his concerns and those of his parents. A good way to start is by encouraging the teen by saying, "Let's try to find a solution" or "Let's look at all the options" or "Let's try to work this out together."

In addition to finding a better solution, we also teach the teen to think and give him models of thinking. We give him feeling of equality and a role in solving his problem in a mature manner. If you create the sense that "we are in this together," it will engender a positive atmosphere. All kinds of suggestions and possible solutions should be written down to consider the consequences of each.

Writing it down makes possible solutions more concrete and easier to discuss. A viable solution should address concerns on both sides and be realistic. Often this initial brainstorming does not elicit many suggestions from the adolescent. The principle of "meeting halfway" teaches flexibility. Each side must give a little to find a solution that both can live with. Trying to find a solution that satisfies both sides will help develop thinking skills. Before a teen can develop this skill, he must learn to ask for help as a way to get a range of ideas and solutions. This is particularly for the adolescent, who is trying to become independent. Pointing out that this is the way adults solve difficult problems may help him to understand it's very unlikely that one person will be able to think of all possibilities and it would be a shame to miss the best solution simply because he didn't think to ask. You can also point out that suggestions from others are not being imposed on him, but rather offered as options to think about.

When a satisfactory solution is found to a problem, it will encourage the teen to ask for help the next time he is confronted with a problem beyond his abilities in the future. The benefit of the CPS approach is that it opens a teen's mind to flexible thinking.

▶ **THE FOURTH STEP IN CPS:**

Select the Best Solution:

Once all solutions are written down by both parent and teen, the final step is to select the best solution. This method allows for full and equal participation of both parties in the process. The most important part of this is to evaluate each solution and reflect on the likely outcome and consequences of each. Once again, this process is very useful to the ADHD teen in terms of learning to develop a long -term outlook. The degree to which each solution is feasible is also very important to review to help teach thinking skills.

Since the ADHD adolescent has limitations in viewing long term consequences, the parent should take the lead in analyzing the possible solutions.

Parent: "If we use this solution, what do you think are the positives and negatives? And if we use solution B, what are the consequences? Which solution do you think is the best for you."

Based on the analysis of the different possibilities, the "best" one should be chosen by the adolescent.

▶ **HOW TO FOLLOW UP IMPLEMENTATION:**

Implementing the solution may require additional support, encouragement and assistance. If there are positive results, the teen should get instant positive feedback. If the teen does not follow up on resolving the problem, then it's time to sit down and discuss what can and should be done. At this stage you should re-evaluate the solution to make sure it is realistic and satisfactory. Encourage him to take the first step. Break down the solution into simpler parts so he can tackle the problem step by step.

Chapter 15

DEVELOP TEAM SPIRIT

▶ **HOW THE NEW APPROACH TO ADHD EMPOWERS PARENTS:**

The new approach to treating the ADHD child enables parents to guide him toward success in life. It is impossible to be effective parents in a state of anger and confusion with no clear direction and guidance. One can acquire the same coaching skills and information and achieve success at a far lower cost with limited professional intervention. The new approach outlined in this book encourages parents to coach a child in life skills. Parents can use daily interactions with their child as an opportunity to give direction and impart emotional and thinking skills. Instead of casual conversations with no purpose or direction, effective communication will enable parents to give their child the training in emotional and thinking skills and guide the child to develop new productive pathways for problem solving. Only parents are in a position to intervene every day as things happen or before a crisis develops.

▶ **WHAT CAN BE DONE IF PARENTS CANNOT ASSUME RESPONSIBILITY?**

The limitation to this new approach is that not all parents are available physically or emotionally to assume the coaching role.

If this is the case, there needs to be a substitute. This could be a grandparent, nanny or someone else who is in daily contact with the child. Parents, older siblings and significant others should all be taught the skills necessary to understand and help the ADHD child. Since a high percentage of parents with ADHD children also have this condition, learning the skills to coach a child can also prove helpful with their own problems. They should get involved with all the CPS and BET exercises with their child.

▶ WHAT IS THE SECRET TO SUCCESS?

1. *Accept your child's condition; don't look for someone to blame.*
Despite the fact that this seems so simple, obvious and natural, it is difficult not to point a finger when it comes to ADHD. There are so many possible sources of blame. One can always blame the teacher, the school system or the crowded classroom. Parents can blame each other by saying that one is too lenient or the other is not home enough. Some parents believe their child is lazy or stubborn. But in order to help the child, parents must accept that the child suffers from a neurological deficit that is beyond anyone's control and must take charge of the treatment to correct it.

2. *Become an expert in CPS and BET.*
This book provides the best information and most recent research in the successful treatment of ADHD. It should give you confidence that with proper medical attention and consistent guidance, most of the symptoms of ADHD can be overcome.

Professional assistance may be necessary from time to time as well as additional training to solve specific issues. However, parents can be a powerful force in helping their child reach his maximum potential.

3. *Implement the new treatment approaches now.*
Many parents say that they do not have the time to deal with treating ADHD. But the implementation of treatment will almost certainly

take less time and be more rewarding than ignoring the problem. It only makes sense that dealing with repetitive crises and conflicts will consume a great deal of time and energy. The impact on the child as well as on the whole family in terms of emotional pain, school problems, and social failures can be quite devastating.

The parent can develop a team mentality, where everyone pitches in to help. That means parents, grandparents, older siblings and caretakers. Families that pull together are happier, more productive and satisfied with their accomplishments.

4. Be tenacious. Patience, persistence and practice will bring success. Keep in mind that parents are not perfect. Practice makes you a better coach. When parents make a mistake, they must be kind and forgiving to themselves. Very few beginnings in any endeavor are things of beauty and grace. Remember the words to the old song, "Pick yourself up, dust yourself off and start all over again." You will "get it" eventually. Two steps forward and one back are normal in the beginning. Don't be hard on yourself or your child. Relax. Take it easy. Lighten up.

Every child is a unique human being; a bit of trial and error before you find the combination of treatments that work best. Praise may be the most potent reinforcement in one child, while for another, a reward system may bring out the best in him. You will find the best combination. No one can know and appreciate a child as much as the parent can. When needed, the parent can seek the advice of professionals and the cooperation of teachers. What job could be more satisfying than molding a wonderful and successful future for one's own child?

The parent should keep track of successes as well as problems and record and date them both. This will be very productive when discussing progress and even problems with the child in the future. With proper medical treatment, collaborative problem solving, and consistent coaching, your child can and will look forward to a successful future.

5. Make sure to get an accurate diagnosis.

The first step is to make sure your child is diagnosed correctly. If there is a learning disability as well as ADHD, this will be revealed with psychological testing. ADHD can only be diagnosed by gathering information and personal history from parents, teachers and significant others. Even though the focus of this book is on therapeutic intervention and collaborative problem solving to ultimately reduce or eliminate the need for medication, it must be emphasized again that methylphenidate is very effective in the treatment of ADHD and dramatically reduces symptoms in most cases. The need to use medication, especially in the beginning or if there is a major crisis, can not be ignored. One must be certain that the optimal dose is being given, as giving too low a dose is ineffective. The results are dramatic and give both the parent and child a calmer environment in which to implement change and learning.

6. Careful planning and organization should be the first order of business.

A 12 year study by several medical centers in the U.S. showed that when medication and proactive therapeutic intervention were used together, the results were significantly better than when medication was given alone. The parent can have a very productive impact on the well being of the child or adolescent by using the collaborative and planning techniques to develop skills that are deficient. The biggest stress in a child's life during the first few years of school is class work and ever increasing expectations. School is the place where ADHD symptoms are most evident and destructive. The teacher may be much less informed than the parent about ADHD and may assume the child is spoiled, self centered, unreasonable, or lazy. The parent may need to educate the teacher and staff and suggest new approaches to help the child or move the child to a different class or school if empathetic and informed professionals are not found. If you are not your child's advocate, it's very likely no one else will be.

7. Begin to record actions, goals and results.
Record specific goals that need to be accomplished in the classroom and evaluate certain behavior patterns once medication and/or therapeutic intervention has begun. Homework assignments need to be carefully monitored. One might need to call the teacher twice a month in the beginning.

8. Focus on your child's needs.
The more consistently one persist with CPS the more one will be rewarded with productive results. Make a list of the conflicts that never seem to be resolved and cause the most serious problems in the child's life. To begin, pick the one that is causing the most difficulty and focus on that. Remember, it is only possible to tackle one problem at a time. Confronting the problem and finding a workable solution will bring a sense of accomplishment and pride from both the parents and the child. In most cases school issues and homework will be top priorities.

9. House rules, Schedule and Organization.
House rules are critical in helping establish a consistent and stable home environment. Develop a regular schedule with the help of the child. This will put order in the child's life and help him to use time efficiently.

   Once the house rules and a schedule of activities are fully implemented, one can move on to establish an effective organized schedule for the child's week. Go with your child to his room to designate the exact place for books, toys, clothes, etc. Insist that he keep his room in order. The lack of clutter and chaos in his room will help him to organize his activities.

10. Solve one problem at a time using CPS.
At this stage, collaborative problem solving can be used to change poor behavior. Your skill as a coach will improve with practice as you deal with problems using this technique. In a like manner,

the child's skills will improve and the parent will work his way out of a job.

The key to successful resolution with this approach is to follow all four steps of CPS. This will allow the child and the parent to overcome specific areas of weakness in either a social or academic nature and insure that the child contributes to the solution to his own problems.

The parent can assist by identifying triggers to precede the unwanted behavior. The longer the list of triggers, the longer will be the list of problems. The parent will slowly reduce the stress and conflict in the child's life as he gains the skills necessary to modulate his emotions, complete his homework, and examine a range of solutions to problems.

11. *Use BET every day.*
The use of brain exercises is very critical to the growth and improvement in mental function. Develop a program to last through childhood and adolescence.

12. *Develop your child's strengths.*
Since the ADHD child compares himself to others his age, he is aware that he is not doing well; homework is harder for him and he is not very successful socially. Often he will try to hide or deny the deficiencies but they are impacting his life every day. Each child has strengths and weaknesses as we all do. To insure that he experiences success and builds self-esteem, the parent can help him find or develop talents and abilities through organized after school activities where he can excel.

Realistic goals can be set that will allow the child to feel a sense of accomplishment. *By accomplishing realistic goals, receiving positive feedback and feeling consistent love, the ADHD child will be able to overcome his challenges.*

For example, the parent could create a project for the child to collect used toys from families in the neighborhood to give to needy children. This goal is simple, can be accomplished in a few days and is realistic. He can feel pride, a sense of accomplishment, and deserving of the praise that his parents will give him.

As has been emphasized, ADHD is a condition where several thinking skills are not fully developed for their age level. Using the CPS approach, executive skills, emotional equilibrium, language development, social skills and cognitive skills can be strengthened. As flexibility in thinking improves and frustration tolerance increases, the level of stress is significantly decreased and the level of confidence and happiness is increased.

These skills will help develop the area of the brain that is deficient in the ADHD child. Remember the old adage: Practice makes perfect. It would be easy to prove a direct correlation between the length of time of practice and skill development in almost any area involving mental function and training for the ADHD child. Make sure the mental exercises are fun. Increasing vocabulary, learning a new language or memorizing facts can all be fun.

13. *Stay on top of the situation.*
One of the benefits of keeping records of meetings, decisions, actions taken, and other pertinent information in a notebook is to be able to review them in black and white with the child at least once a week. It makes the issues more concrete. Progress in school, in social situations and at home can be reviewed together. This is a good time to open communication with the child to make sure there are not issues troubling him that have been missed. Review the house rules and the schedule to re-enforce the commitment to adhere to both. Use this weekly review to focus on the positive and don't miss a single opportunity to praise your child. This can be the most valuable time spent with the child all week.

14. *Use effective complimentary methods.*
After being cleared by a medical check up, there is no reason why

medication can not be extremely beneficial since it literally corrects the neurotransmitter deficit, just as giving insulin compensates for the pancreas not producing enough insulin in a diabetic. While it does not make permanent changes in the brain, Ritalin restores normal function and may facilitate the implementation of BET and CPS as well as other strategies. An adolescent who has not been diagnosed earlier will usually benefit from medication during the time before enhanced brain development through all the strategies we have discussed.

Regular vigorous physical exercise has been shown to be very beneficial and should be done at least 40 minutes five days a week in adolescents. Aerobic exercise is Nature's brain tonic. The brain is washed in cleansing agents, nutrients, growth factors, oxygen, neurotropic agents and other beneficial substances. Organized sports have many social benefits. Jump rope, fast walking, running in place, etc. are also effective, although not as effective as exercise that involves strategy. Vigorous exercise just before homework, has been shown to aid concentration and focus just as it does in younger children. In addition, just before bed, incorporate a number of balance exercises. Experiment to see what works best for your child. This needs to be done at least five days a week to have a significant impact on the child's behavior, mood and thinking skills. The parent can help to incorporate these new activities in a natural and enjoyable way. Get a narrow board, raise it a foot or two above the ground and make a game emphasizing balance. After mastering the board, get one that is even narrower.

15. *Make as many activities as possible family affairs.*

Food and Supplements:
If a child eats a balanced diet every day, vitamin supplements are not necessary. In the real world, few children eat a fully balanced diet. Vitamin and mineral supplements should be taken as needed.

Fish and flax seed Omega 3 were found to help in the reduction of the severity of ADHD symptoms.

In the kitchen, try to avoid the use of additives and to lower the sugar content in the child's diet. Empty calories are not beneficial and your child may be sensitive to some additives.

Relaxation:
A child can use relaxation techniques when he feels overwhelmed or about to lose control. Remind him to use them whenever he feels frustrated or angry.

Learn to take care of yourself:
Parents cannot be effective if they are unhappy. Find activities that are enjoyable and meaningful. Accentuate the positive in life and concentrate on aspects of life that engender pride/happiness/satisfaction. Live a healthy life style with generous amounts of exercise, proper diet and rest. Develop a hobby or join a social group with similar interests to expand horizons.

One should cherish and nurture the relationship with one's spouse. Have a regular time each week just for each other and plan to spend a long weekend just for fun and enjoyment away from the responsibilities of family. Nurture meaningful friendships as they are a source of strength and help.

Exercise regularly:
Exercise is the best way to boost stamina and endurance as well as contribute to a healthy life style. Combine exercise with socializing by finding friends who are also interested in a regular exercise program.

Give yourself a treat:
After a hard week, try to have an activity that is particularly enjoyable. Maybe a massage, a musical event, or a hobby will give you that extra boost of enjoyment. Make sure there are events

in the schedule that are really enjoyable. There's no need to be a martyr.

Learn How to Reduce Stress:
In addition to all the above, share the household responsibilities evenly. Both parents must share the household and parenting responsibilities so that one is not overwhelmed. Older children should have specific responsibilities as well.

Learn to Express Yourself:
Begin to tactfully say what is on your mind. Do not keep frustration, anger or disappointment inside. Keep in mind that you need to be responsible in your expression of feelings and avoid blame.

Relaxation Exercises for the Mom:
Relaxation techniques tend to lower stress levels. Progressive muscle relaxation involving deep breathing, yoga or other techniques can keep anger and frustration in perspective.

Gratitude for all the good things in life should be a daily routine.

Concentrate on these aspects of your life before going to sleep at night and make them your first thoughts in the morning.

In conclusion, keep everything in perspective. Overcoming ADHD is one of many challenges of life. It's a minor glitch in the most complex organ, the human brain, and can be treated effectively. Children with ADHD can display high intelligence, astonishing creativity, amazing intuition, artistic talent and charisma. Be happy for all the wonderful qualities that make your child a special, unique person. Enjoy your time together, don't be discouraged, and keep a positive attitude.

▶ **IMPORTANT POINTS TO REMEMBER:**

- A parent able to coach his child can help him to overcome his symptoms and achieve success.
- A full program needs to be planned and implemented if not by the parent, then by another adult who will be willing to consistently work to implement the program.
- This new approach has many components that can be integrated and adapted to each family situation.
- Proper diagnosis and full medical evaluation is a must before one starts the new approach.
- The heart and soul of the new approach is CPS and BET.
- Each parent/coach can become skilled in using CPS and BET. They can develop all the professional skills needed to help their child.
- To see permanent changes and relief from symptoms, these two techniques and other strategies need to be used for several years but you will see steady improvement.
- Medication can be decreased or even eliminated as the symptoms diminish over the course of treatment.

Chapter 16

ADULTS WITH ADHD

While there are many examples of famous personalities who proved highly successful despite suffering from ADHD without treatment, statistically, untreated adult ADHD cases are less promising. Just as everyone knows of an individual who smoked a pack of cigarettes a day and a lived to be 100, it's wise to consider the reality of the broader population. For ADHD, the statistics are sobering. There is much higher divorce rate for ADHD sufferers, a higher rater of occupational failure, many more accidents and financial mismanagement. This is the reality.

During my years as an assistant professor of psychiatry and as co-director with my wife at the Marriage and Sex Counseling Clinic in the medical school at Emory University, we saw many couples across a socio-economic spectrum.

When ADHD symptoms were present in the behavior of a husband and/or wife, dysfunction would typically appear in many areas, from family to work to social relationships. Family dysfunction was reflected in poor financial planning, workaholic lifestyles, disrupted relationships and poor communication. In the work place, frequent job changes or poor job performance was typical. This isn't to say that every person with adult ADHD will manifest *all* the symptoms. Many people with ADHD unconsciously seek conflict. The urge for novelty and impulsivity often combine to create turmoil even when other symptoms seem mild.

In treatment, the husband and wife usually speak privately with a therapist before beginning couples therapy. This is a summary of a typical scenario for a couple in which the husband has ADHD: Jennifer: "I know Max loves our children and me but I feel like we live from crisis to crisis. I've lost track of the number of jobs he's held, even though he's very talented in his field. We fight a lot about money. I learned by accident that our life insurance policy had expired and we seem to be overdrawn all the time with no savings whatsoever. He is very cavalier about these kinds of things, which drives me crazy. Caring for our two teenagers is primarily my responsibility because he can not deal with the problems of adolescents without losing his temper.

Our social life is also very limited. He's a workaholic and it's not easy for him to establish friendships. Sometimes people are offended by his sense of humor, or he forgets appointments and leaves friends waiting. There's a long list of minor social blunders that are, each individually, not a big deal. But together they form a pattern that does not encourage relaxed friendships. I know he loves us and he's really a good person but our marriage is suffering."

Max: "My wife insisted that we come here. I know we have some problems, but so do most couples. I work very hard to support my family and they are the main focus in my life. I do have trouble meeting deadlines at work and always seem be running behind. I come home frustrated, tense and exhausted. I've had a problem with organization for as long as I can remember. Thank goodness I have a very high energy level and can usually compensate for this by working longer and harder.

As far as our two teenage boys are concerned, I leave most of the discipline up to my wife because I cannot seem to control my temper. I know my wife is unhappy with the way things are, but I don't know what to do about it."

In this case, it was important to bring the whole family together. The parents were advised to plan activities such as hiking and camping out. Marriage counseling included developing organizational skills, improving communication and parenting skills and developing intimacy as well as shared friendships.

Money matters were turned over to a financial planner. Max worked on improving his parenting skills and developing common interests with his sons. The parents reported greater satisfaction with their marriage and agreed to "touch base'" whenever needed. The husband and wife began a vigorous exercise program and even yoga classes together.

ADHD symptoms present in many different ways in adults. The following is an example of infidelity impacting a marriage:

Anne: "We've been married almost 20 years in October. Although we love each other, I'm not happy. We seem to be drifting apart, but I can't put my finger on the problem. Our life together feels so chaotic. We've moved three times in the past five years because James always sees greener pastures just over the hill. He's a very talented salesman, so he's always in demand. But because of all the anxiety, our sex life is almost non-existent. We seem to be going through the motions of every day living.

My work is very satisfying and challenging. Without that outlet, I would be very depressed."

James: "I'm worried I'm losing my wife. I know she's not happy and I have a lot of guilt about that because I know I'm not the best husband in the world.

Therapist: What do you think are the main issues?

James: "I know so many moves have taken a toll. It's an adjustment for her and for the kids. She's a wonderful mother. I'm amazed at how easy it is for her to deal with our teenagers. I don't have the patience."

Therapist: "Do you think the moves are the cause of her unhappiness?"

James: "No." (silent)

"With every move I seem to start up a new affair. It's always with someone in the office, which could endanger my job. I know I am risking my marriage, my job and my reputation, but I can't seem to help myself. With each move, I tell myself it won't happen again. It usually starts because I can't seem to meet deadlines or I miss appointments. One of the girls in the office is assigned to assist me after hours and it goes from there. I love my wife and don't want to lose her. She's my best friend.

I know that sounds phony, but I can't seem to resist the excitement of the affair. Afterwards, I feel nothing but guilt and remorse. I think sometimes the affairs are a substitute for my lack of advancement at work. I have anxiety all the time about papers I've misplaced, business cards I can't find or opportunities I've screwed up. I know I can not move up to a management position when I can't organize my own professional agenda and my personal life is in such a mess".

The risky behavior, impulsive job changes, a serious lack of organizational skills as well as professional advancement below his ability level are classic adult ADHD symptoms. Further investigation would reveal numerous driving violations, an inability to relax and a serious lack of planning for the future.

The lack of treatment for so many years compromised almost every aspect of his life. Ritalin was prescribed and marriage counseling recommended. Although BET and CPS were not developed forms of therapy at that time, marriage counseling incorporated many aspects of CPS and the couple was coached to work on improving their communication, social skills and problem solving techniques.

We discovered quite by accident that in many cases, vigorous exercise was beneficial and a regular exercise program was implemented for both husband and wife. Marriage counseling continued once a week for over 18 months to improve communication skills, enhance intimacy and to deal with problems as they developed. For the next three years, individual counseling was necessary for James. Once he understood the cause of his risky behavior, we were able to work on new methods of coping with stress, developing problem-solving techniques and enhancing his organizational, skills step by step. Insight into a reason for his affairs helped him to develop other coping mechanisms, James's promiscuous behavior ceased. Communication, intimacy and trust developed rapidly, partly because the couple was highly motivated to save the marriage and partly because they understood the main reason for their difficulties.

Though the theory of brain plasticity was not understood at the time this couple sought therapy, many techniques used in therapy utilized aspects of CPS and BET, simply because they were found to be effective.

A summary of a session with an ADHD wife:

Linda: "I am overwhelmed at work. I've been promoted to a new position with much more responsibility. I was barely able to perform as things were, and now, I just don't know what to do. I can't manage the kids at all. They are wild and out of control. I feel depressed and anxious all the time. I'm so consumed at work that I don't have any emotional reserves. I usually come home late and exhausted. I can't stand to fail, but the work is overwhelming. The demands my husband makes and his complaints just make me feel guilty and depressed."

Therapist: "Do you remember other times in your life when you felt this way?"

Linda: "Oh yes. I dreaded school for as long as I can remember. I could never concentrate and was known as a disorganized kid. Fortunately, my parents were well off enough to get tutors for me or I would never have made it through high school. College was stressful too. I constantly lost or didn't finish my assignments. I managed to get my act together enough to finish college with mediocre grades. During this time, I discovered that I have abilities in salesmanship and that has carried me professionally.

I think I "sold" my husband on the idea of marrying me. He probably regrets it.

I am absolutely useless when it comes to dealing with the kids. I don't have the patience."

Therapist: "Why have you come for help now?"

Linda: "The crisis that brought us here has to do with our sex life. I would not be surprised to learn that my husband is having an affair. He is fed up and hurt by my behavior. I love him so much and I know he would find that hard to believe right now. I have been very depressed since my promotion and feel guilty that I am such a failure as a wife and mother and even as a friend. I don't know what to do. I can't seem to help myself."

Mark: "I have been thinking of divorce. My wife is hard to live with. She is so involved with her work that the kids and I are pretty much on our own. Often she doesn't come home until 9 p.m. and even then, she just collapses into bed. I am naturally a very affectionate and extroverted person and usually very optimistic and easy going. I love being with people and have many friends. I can say that most of our friends are really my friends. My wife does not have many social outlets. But that's not the main issue.

I feel rejected. Our sex life is terrible. In fact, our life together in general is suffering. My wife has many wonderful qualities. She's very creative and kind. We married very young and used to have a lot of fun together. Now I can't remember the last time we really enjoyed being together.

Linda loves me, and I know that. But I'm not willing to live the rest of my life like this. I find myself drawn to other women, although I haven't had an affair. Divorce would be terrible for our kids and is almost unheard of in my family. If things don't change, I will probably stick it out until they are in college. I know our situation has to change for our marriage to last, but right now we are just going through the motions."

Further testing revealed ADHD in Linda and one of her children. This diagnosis was life changing. Ritalin was prescribed in the beginning of treatment. She was encouraged to discuss her situation with her superior. Once there was understanding, her boss assigned an assistant to help her relieve some of her chronic pressure. She began an aerobic exercise program, which not only relieved her ADHD symptoms, but increased her endurance. We made regular exercise part of the family agenda. The child with ADHD was also included. Developing problem-solving techniques and communication skills were top priorities. Marriage counseling continued once a week for over 10 months and after that was reduced to twice monthly and finally once a month over the next year.

▸ WHAT RISK FACTORS CONTRIBUTE TO THE PERSISTENCE OF ADHD INTO ADULTHOOD?

Three risk factors contribute to the persistence of ADHD into adult life. Studies by Beiderman in 1995 suggest that as many as 50% of the children diagnosed with ADHD have symptoms that persist into adulthood. Although ADHD symptoms vary in degree, a decline in hyperactivity and impulsive behavior is typical as a child becomes an adult, while inattention and lack of focus often persist. The three risk factors that have been identified as having the most impact of the possibility a child with ADHD continuing to have symptoms into adulthood:

(1) Family history of ADHD

(2) The presence of associated (i.e. depression, alcohol and drug use, conduct disorder, learning disabilities)

(3) Psychological adversity: Examples would be a mother who has similar difficulties or is ineffective at setting boundaries, a depressed mother or a mother who can not show consistent stable support to the ADHD child.

► WHAT IS THE SIGNIFICANCE OF THESE RISK FACTORS?

The ADHD child with only one of these risk factors has a 20% chance of his symptoms persisting into adulthood. A child with two of the above risk factors early in life has a 30% chance of continued symptoms, while all three risk factors raise the probability to 70%.

Knowing the significance of these risk factors can help adults suffering from this condition and reduce the chance of their children carrying with these symptoms into adulthood. The prevalence of ADHD in adults has been estimated at 4% of the general population. However because of the relatively recent emergence of Adult ADHD as a diagnosis, the condition probably remains under-diagnosed and untreated in adults.

► HOW DOES FAILURE TO LEARN FROM THE PAST IMPACT ADULT ADHD?

The consequences of not learning from the past or preparing effectively for the future will express itself in very concrete ways. Many adults will not have a savings plans or medical insurance. They may not plan for retirement or work to develop financial stability for the family. More commonly, the ADHD adult will live from crisis to crisis without foreseeing approaching events. This lack of foresight can have disastrous consequences; missed deadlines, broken promises, forgotten appointments are only a few of the results. Serious marital conflicts and constant family stress are another. When a couple tells me that one of the main issues that are a source of marital conflict is money, I always investigate further for ADHD as a possible cause.

► HOW DO UNTREATED SYMPTOMS COMPOUND THE PROBLEM?

For most ADHD adults, the inability to anticipate and plan for the future causes them to feel inadequate, depressed and even helpless. It contributes to a high degree of depression, alcohol abuse and anti-social behavior. All of the above combined with family conflicts and poor interaction with children can easily lead to separation or divorce.

Many adults with ADHD are heavy smokers, abuse drugs and alcohol, drive carelessly, gamble or take other risks. This behavior is often an attempt to reduce the stress and frustration of their symptoms. All of these risky activities demonstrate that most adults with ADHD suffer from the consequences of their condition without any understanding of its etiology or the availability of treatment.

▶ DO ASSOCIATED CONDITIONS OF ANXIETY / DEPRESSION LEAD TO FUNCTIONAL IMPAIRMENT?

About 80% of adult ADHD will exhibit associated conditions such as depression.

Many adults with ADHD experience one or more major depressions during adult life.

About 35% of both males and females report a period of major depression. Anxiety is the most prevalent condition associated with adult ADHD. As many as 50% of adults report anxiety symptoms without a specific cause.

There's a commonality for:

Isaac, a 37 year old high level executive, reported a high degree of restlessness, poor sleep patterns, and feelings of anxiety and depression when he reported to the clinic. He stated that these feelings commonly emerge when his company sends him out of town for a week of training. Though the training usually paves the way to a promotion and higher pay, the fear of the exam at the end of the training is a source of stress. When asked about previous educational experiences, he stated that the worst time of his life was during high school. He barely graduated and actually had to drop out of college. However, his computer skills and sales capabilities allowed him to progress in his company. When a careful history was taken of his childhood, ADHD symptoms were prevalent. Additional testing and a self-rating confirmed the ADHD diagnosis for the first time.

In Susan's case, she arrived at the clinic complaining of feeling blue for the past few months. A 32 year-old mother of two children aged 2 and 5, she cried easily and frequently, had a poor appetite and could not sleep at night. She stopped calling her friends and even felt distant from her mother. She was able to get a leave of absence from her job just before she started a new position there. She stated that since her husband is spending a lot more time out of town, many more responsibilities had fallen on her shoulders. Her five-year-old seemed out of control and the demands of her job were increasing. In short, she felt she could not cope with these new demands. It was determined that her ability to plan and organize her life was poor and now with her husband unavailable, she could not function effectively. She reported having difficulty with concentration most of her life, a short temper and often not finishing what she started. However, she kept busy all the time because it took so long to accomplish each task.

As in the previous case history, the associated depression was the main concern. Untreated depression can lead to serious consequences. Like Isaac, Susan was never diagnosed as having ADHD in the past. She was able to compensate in different ways until the demands placed upon her outstripped her capacity to deal effectively with them.

Learning Disabilities:

Many adults with ADHD will continue to suffer throughout life from learning disabilities. These adults avoid reading and most careers that require heavy reading, such as law, academics and medicine. Even a long list of instructions is enough to put them off a new piece of equipment. Most are overwhelmed by their combined handicaps.

► **HOW ARE ADULTS WITH ADHD IMPACTED BY DRUGS AND ALCOHOL?**

Marshall, a 47-year-old male, arrived in my office a day after his boss threatened to fire him over his drinking. Marshall, a successful vice-president of a large public company, appeared agitated and restless.

Marshall: "I'm afraid that I'm going to lose my job. I started as a local sales representative 10 years ago and did so well that I was promoted to vice president of marketing and sales. Now, I may lose it all. It would be very hard for me to start over. Even though I make over $250,000 a year, I'm always in debt. My boss made it clear that if I don't stop drinking, he will fire me. I'm a great earner for the company, but I know he's serious."

Therapist: "Was there any specific event that led up to this statement?"

Marshall: "Yes. Last week I was out of town for a regional meeting. I was nervous about the presentation I had to give on a new line of products. I was given a lot of reading material about the new products only a few days earlier. The president asked me to present the material for the first time. I was overwhelmed and to calm down, I drank. I began drinking the night before the presentation and by the next day I was so drunk I couldn't leave my hotel room. Fortunately, my two assistants were able to do the presentation for me, but that evening I got a call from my boss telling me to come to his office the next day. It was not the first time I turned to alcohol when faced with pressure. I drink regularly to keep my anxiety down and clear my head. However, when there is increased pressure and demands on me, I drink more with the hope that it will reduce my anxiety.

I keep a full work schedule of more than 12 hours a day and I get good results. A lot of my company's success is due to my sales capabilities. My boss recognizes my poor organizational skills and planning, so I'm always given extra time to complete my tasks. My family life suffers because of my work schedule and my drinking. I love my children and my wife but I know I spend very little time at home. I just don't know how to deal with all my responsibilities."

Therapist: "When did you start to drink?"

Marshall: "At around 14. Drugs and alcohol helped me function better. College life was very difficult. I was simply not able to do the academic work. I am not sure whether the drinking or the poor academic performance caused me to quit college. I always seemed to turn to alcohol when faced with a challenge. Maybe it helps me stay calmer, but it has a terrible effect on my life."

Therapist: "You said you had difficulties during high school. Do you recall any problems in grade school?"

Marshall: "During grammar school I spent more time in the hallway than I did in class. I just couldn't sit still. I seldom finished my homework on time and every small distraction ruined my concentration."

Therapist: "It seems that homework and school in general was very stressful.

Marshall: Absolutely!"

Marshall was given the Adult Self-Rating Scale which, together with additional information, helped make the ADHD diagnosis.

▶ **IS THE RATE OF SMOKING HIGHER AMONG ADHD ADULTS?**

There is a high rate of nicotine use with adult ADHD. More than 50% of adults with ADHD smoke heavily. Many studies point to the fact that nicotine enhances concentration and attention. This may explain why, under stress, ADHD adults increase their tobacco intake significantly.

We have new propelling evidence that nicotine causes ADHD. One is that a mother who smokes during pregnancy increases the risk that her baby will have ADHD. Up to 22% of mothers who smoke bear children with some degree of ADHD.

In the general smoking population, 48% are able to successfully quit smoking. Only 29% of ADHD individuals who smoke are able to quit. Caffeine also seems to have some calming influence on the restless ADHD adult. Self-medication with cigarettes and excessive coffee drinking are often overlooked by therapists and doctors, but may actually be the first clue to the presence of ADHD.

Another form of dangerous self-medication is drug abuse. Untreated ADHD adults are more likely to indulge in risky behavior up to the age of 50. There appear to be two peaks in drug use – during the late twenties and again in the late forties. By the time the untreated ADHD adult reaches his fifties, as many as 55% may be using drugs. Earlier in adult life, the rate is much lower.

▶ HOW SERIOUS IS OPPOSITIONAL DEFIANT DISORDER IN ADULTS?

Often adolescent ODD seems to be resolved by the time the teen enters adult years. However, a high percentage of adolescents who exhibit conduct disorder during their teen years have continued conduct disorder symptoms as adults. Studies show that about 50% of this group continue to develop serious anti-social behavior. A study of the prison population in the U.S. in 1994 shows that about 25% of the inmate population was diagnosed with ADHD. This condition should be given full attention by authorities and remedial steps taken.

▶ WHAT ARE THE MAJOR FUNCTIONAL IMPAIRMENTS OF ADULT ADHD?

Many adults whose underlying difficulty is ADHD often complain not only of depression, work and family conflicts but also of difficulty in dealing with their children.

Of course, if a child also has ADHD, the problem is magnified. Occupational failure, social and intellectual deficits as well as family conflict will top the list of functional impairments that the adult with ADHD faces all his life.

▶ HOW DO ADULT ADHD SYMPTOMS IMPACT JOB PERFORMANCE?

Since adults with ADHD experience similar symptoms to children with ADHD, the manifestation of these symptoms will reflect the changes in their activities and responsibilities.

The restless feelings experienced in childhood can appear to be sheer ambition. As adults they are constantly on the go and are often described as workaholics. Being hyperactive attracts them to jobs in fields such as sales and marketing that are more dynamic than some of the alternatives.

Sometimes adults with ADHD try to do two jobs at once, working long hours or selecting a job that requires physical effort. On the other hand, many ADHD symptoms lead to serious work related problems. Failing to complete tasks, especially if the tasks are routine, can cause conflicts with supervisors and coworkers.

The Milwaukee Young Adult Study in 2002 found that adults with ADHD are more than twice as likely to be fired from their job as other workers. They display more oppositional defiant disorder on the job and have lower work performance rating from supervisors. They are twice as likely to change jobs as their peers. Because of low frustration tolerance, they exhibit explosive irritable behavior toward supervisors and coworkers and frequently end up in conflict. They constantly look for a better, different job and as a result, many ADHD adults have difficulty finding and keeping a job and their job performance is below the level of their competence. Despite similar educational levels and IQ scores, adults with ADHD display lower occupational accomplishment as a group.

A small group of ADHD adults with anti-social personality disorder act out to the extent that they are fired. The majority of ADHD adults find themselves in serious conflict with their supervisors at some point. They have few skills to prevent the consequences. Many of the poor performance problems related to completion of tasks in the work place are caused by failure in organization, planning and time management. This, along with poor social skills, seems to be the main causes of job stress.

▶ WHAT TYPES OF PROFESSIONS ARE BEST SUITED TO ADHD ADULTS?

Many of the successful ADHD adults are able to find positions that allow them to capitalize on their strengths and minimize their deficiencies. Working in a position with less supervision allows them to express their strengths and capabilities with minimum interference. Jobs in TV and radio, acting, sports, entertainment and computer programming are examples. Work in sales or marketing, where specific goals are clearly defined with time limits, help the adult with ADHD function better. Working independently in any field of interest may minimize friction and conflict.

▶ WHAT ARE THE CONSEQUENCES OF ADULT ADHD SYMPTOMS ON EDUCATION?

Just like high school, higher education is problematic for the ADHD sufferer. The drop out rate is four times higher. Suspension as well as expulsions is three times higher than the average student. As a group, educational and vocational performance is below average based on the person's intelligence and education.

▶ WHAT IS THE IMPACT OF ADULT ADHD SYMPTOMS ON FAMILY LIFE?

The impact of adult ADHD symptoms on family life can lead to serious family conflict and enough stress to lead to divorce. Since the likelihood that adults with ADHD will have a child with a similar condition is around 50%, parenting difficulties will trigger constant conflict. It is difficult for an ADHD parent to implement many of the treatment goals for the ADHD child. Their poor organization, lack of frustration tolerance and inability to provide guidance, leadership and supervision will almost certainly lead to friction and failure despite sincere efforts. Poor money management and failure to take care of financial matters like paying bills, completing tax returns, or maintaining active insurance policies will compound spousal conflicts and chaos in family life. Poor listening skills, impulsive comments, and inadequate social skills add to the negative atmosphere. All of these deficiencies have a serious impact on family life. Effective treatment of the adult with ADHD can greatly reduce, if not eliminate, this debilitating condition and reduce conflict to a minimum.

▶ **WHAT IS THE IMPACT OF ADULT ADHD ON PERSONAL RELATIONSHIPS?**

Adults with ADHD have had to cope with their symptoms for years. They have had time to develop compensatory mechanisms to minimize the impact of their symptoms on their life. However, really understanding the etiology of ADHD can help correct the neurological deficit rather than creating elaborate coping mechanisms to mask the impairment.

Friendships are often difficult. The tendency to express anger quickly, comment impulsively, and overlook the needs of others are not helpful in building and maintaining friendships. Because of these poor interpersonal skills (Barkley and Murphy 2000), they will have few means with which to nurture and sustain friendships. Understanding and recognizing these poorly developed skills will be the first step in correcting these impairments.

▶ **WHAT ARE THE FACTORS LEADING TO RISKY BEHAVIOR?**

Risky behavior complicates and seriously impairs functioning. It is not only the relatively small anti-social group within the adult ADHD population that engages in highly risky behavior. A check of official driving records reveals that the ADHD group had many more citations for speeding, more license suspensions and more crashes than non-ADHD adults.

There is a marked increase in gambling as well as other

addictive behavior. The high degree of risky behavior by adults with ADHD is attributed to inadequate levels of dopamine in the brain, according to Dr. Velkow, M.D. Engaging in risky activities increases the level of this neurotransmitter and calms the adult with ADHD. Proper treatment can lower or even eliminate the urge to pursue this behavior.

▶ **WHAT IS THE MIND-BODY CONNECTION?**

Harvard professor Dr. Tal Ben-Shachar puts it this way: "I explain to my students that there is a connection between body and mind. Studies show that doing physical exercise three times a week for half an hour each time has the same effect as Zolof, a powerful anti-depressant... human nature is not built for sitting in front of the TV or computer screens all day... and if you don't give the body what it wants, you pay a price."

▶ **IMPORTANT POINTS TO REMEMBER:**

- As many as 50% of children diagnosed with ADHD will have some of their symptoms persist into adult life.
- Adult ADHD symptoms vary in frequency of occurrence, pervasiveness and degree of severity.
- About 4% of the general adult population exhibits ADHD symptoms.
- Family history, the presence of associated conditions like depression, alcohol abuse, or psychological adversities, increase the risk of persistent symptoms in adult life.
- The rate of smoking among adults with ADHD is twice as high as the general population and it is much harder for them to quit.
- High rates of drug and alcohol abuse among adults with ADHD contribute to the high percentage of oppositional defiant disorder and anti-social behavior in the group.
- Adult ADHD symptoms can lead to major impairment in family life, the work place, and academic performance.

- Adult ADHD can lead to risky behavior, inappropriate sexual relationships, and anti-social activity.
- Adults with ADHD can embrace the steps that will improve relationships, upgrade their job performance and enhance the quality of their lives.

Chapter 17

DIAGNOSING ADULT ADHD

$\mathbf{D}$r. Daniel Amen, a neuroscientist and psychiatrist, discusses one of his cases in his book, "Change Your Brain, Change Your Life."

Sally, a 40-year-old woman, had been hospitalized under his care for depression, anxiety and suicidal thoughts. "In my clinical interview with her, I discovered that she had many adult ADD symptoms (such as short attention span, distractibility, disorganization and restlessness). She had a son with ADD (a frequent tip to diagnosing ADD in adults). Despite her IQ of 140, she had never finished college, and she was employed below her ability as a laboratory technician. "I decided to order a SPECT study on Sally." (A SPECT scan involves injecting radioactive isotopes to measure metabolic brain activity.) "Sally's brain activity was abnormal. At rest, she had good overall brain activity, especially in the prefrontal cortex. But when she was asked to perform math problems (an exercise to challenge her ability to concentrate), she had marked decreased activity across her whole brain, especially in the prefrontal cortex. I placed her on a low dose of Ritalin. She had a wonderful response. Her mood was better, she was less anxious, and she could concentrate for longer periods of time.

She eventually went back to school and finished her degree. No longer did she think of herself as an underachiever, but rather as someone who needs treatment for a medical problem." She said, "Having ADD is not my fault. It's a medical problem, just like someone who needs glasses."

► **WHAT ARE THE CRITERIA FOR DIAGNOSING ADHD?**

Adult ADHD was recognized as a medical condition for the first time in 1994.

The American Psychiatric Association established the full criteria to diagnose adult ADHD.

Criteria for Predominantly Inattentive Type of ADHD:

Six or more of the following must be manifested often:

- Inattention to details; careless mistakes
- Difficulty sustaining attention
- Seems not to listen
- Fails to finish tasks
- Difficulty organizing
- Avoids tasks requiring sustained attention
- Loses things
- Easily distracted
- Forgetful

Criteria for Predominantly Hyperactive-Impulsive Type of ADHD:

Six or more of the following manifested often:

- Impulsivity
- Blurts out answer before question is finished
- Difficulty awaiting turn
- Interrupts or intrudes on others
- Hyperactivity
- Fidgets
- Unable to stay seated
- Inappropriate restlessness
- Difficulty with quiet leisure activities

- On the go
- Talks incessantly

▶ **WHAT ARE THE CONDITIONS REQUIRED TO MAKE THE DIAGNOSIS?**

Symptoms of inattention, impulsivity/hyperactivity that:
- Have persisted for more than 6 months and are severe and frequent
- Onset of symptoms prior to age 7
- Causes severe impairment in 2 or more settings
- Causes significant impairment in social academic or occupational functioning
- Are not better accounted for by another diagnosis

▶ **SUBTYPES OF ADULT ADHD:**

ADHD Predominantly Inattentive Type
- Criteria are met for inattention but not for impulsivity/hyperactivity

ADHD Predominantly Hyperactive/Impulsive Type
- Criteria are met for impulsivity/hyperactivity but not inattention

ADHD Combined Type
- Criteria are met for both inattention and impulsivity/hyperactivity

ADHD not otherwise specified:
- Full criteria are not met; unclear whether criteria have been met in the past.

▶ **WHAT DOES IT TAKE TO MAKE THE DIAGNOSIS?**

Studies showed that only 10% of adults with ADHD will function normally. About 30 % will overcome about half their symptoms and about 60% will have a marked decrease in their initial symptoms that caused them difficulty in normal functioning. Just like children and adolescents, evaluation of adult ADHD remains a clinical diagnosis requiring a careful clinical evaluation with an accurate history.

Current symptoms and functional impairment need to be analyzed along with historical information about childhood onset of symptoms. In addition, other medical disorders must be eliminated as a possible cause of the symptoms. The use of rating scales will be helpful to clarify and quantify some of the symptoms. The actual evaluation of adults with ADHD is not simple. Adults have usually developed numerous, sometimes elaborate, compensatory mechanisms to cope with their deficiencies.

► **CAN YOU RECOGNIZE THE SYMPTOMS OF ADULT ADHD?**

The key symptoms of inattention, hyperactivity and impulsivity may be manifested in adult life in different forms. Symptoms of restlessness may be transformed into workaholic adults. A child who is excessively active may become an adult with a job that emphasizes physical or risky activity. A child that cannot stay seated may over-schedule with meetings and be overwhelmed with work constraints as an adult.

A child that is "on the go" may manifest symptoms as an adult of being involved in constant activity such as sports, clubs, hobbies, etc. to the detriment of his family. Adult symptoms of impulsivity may manifest themselves as low frustration tolerance, irritation, and difficulty with co-workers and in social settings. Unfortunately, this is also expressed in driving behavior. Driving too fast, running red lights or stop signs, and 'road rage' are all repressed impulsive behavior or loss of focus. In the job setting, quitting because of minor conflicts or frustration, difficulty with co-workers or frequent job changes may be symptoms of ADHD. In personal relationships, ending relationships suddenly or making impulsive commitments, are symptoms of ADHD. Symptoms of inattention often manifest differently in adults as well. Reading is limited and extensive tasks will result in paralyzing procrastination. The easily distractible and forgetful child will be a disorganized, forgetful adult who has difficulty with planning and execution and completing tasks.

▶ **WHAT ARE THE CRITERIA FOR A DEFINITIVE DIAGNOSIS OF ADULT ADHD?**

For complete and accurate diagnosis of adult ADHD, six of the nine symptoms of both the inattention and impulsivity/hyperactivity symptoms must be present. The second criterion is impairment in two separate settings – academic, work, family or social. For most adults, family and job impairment will be prominent. Relationships with wife and children are usually the first to be affected. Constant fights and disagreements about child rearing, household responsibilities, and money matters usually head the list. The list will include shared responsibilities, communication, and emotional and sexual dissatisfaction. Impairment at the work place will manifest itself in frequent job changes, conflict with supervisors and co-workers, failing to complete tasks and being fired. In academic or vocational settings, the adult with ADHD will find many difficulties in completing required academic work. Identifying two separate areas of significant impairment is an essential part of the adult ADHD diagnosis.

The final requirement to complete the diagnosis is to verify that some of the symptoms date back to early childhood. To complete childhood history, information should be obtained from parents or older siblings when possible. Formal records from grade school can be useful.

▶ **HOW USEFUL IS THE SELF-RATING SCALE FOR DIAGNOSING ADULT ADHD?**

To help determine that symptoms are not due to a lack of effort or other medical conditions, the use of self-rating scales can be very useful. Use of rating scales will help determine whether other diagnoses should be considered or whether other associated conditions are impacting the symptoms and impairments.

Use of Adult ADHD Scales:

Rating scales are helpful in assessing whether an individual meets the diagnostic criteria of Adult ADHD. Rating scales provide the structure to assess current symptoms and their severity. They can complement and validate the presence of at least six of the DSM IV symptoms to establish valid and reliable diagnoses of adult ADHD.

▶ **WHAT ARE SOME OF THE ADULT SELF-RATING SCALES (ASRS)?**

There are several diagnostic systems and rating scales that provide symptom assessment. Functional impairment in occupational or social arenas are important features of ADHD but are not specific to ADHD.

The Conner's Adult ADHD Diagnostic Interview for DSM IV is a clinician- administered interview that assesses the presence of the 18 DSM-IV symptoms for children and adults. Impairments at school, work, home and in social settings are evaluated from childhood to adulthood.

Questions about childhood history, difficulties during pregnancy and delivery, temperament, development, medical and risk factors are investigated. Childhood academic history as well as adult educational and psychiatric background are investigated. Finally there is screening for associated conditions such as learning disabilities. This diagnostic interview scale is one of the most popular and used by many professionals.

Other diagnostic scales include Barkley's Current Symptoms Scale Self-Report and Brown's ADD Scale Diagnostic Form. The rating scale that is used most frequently is The Current Symptoms Surveys. This scale can be divided into clinician-administered and self-reported forms.

The following tests are used to identify specific areas of weakness and can help clinicians understand how the patient processes different types of information. They are useful when trying to identify executive dysfunction (the ability to make and execute plans, evaluation, decision making) or diagnose learning disorders.

▶ **WISC-III:**

The Wechsler Individual Achievement test (WISC) and WISC-III are commonly used. WISC-III allows for meaningful analysis of ability and achievement. Discrepancies in the verbal and non-verbal part of the test are used in the diagnosis of learning disabilities.

It employs eight sub-tests involving:
(1) Basic reading
(2) Math
(3) Spelling
(4) Reading comprehension
(5) Numerical operations
(6) Listening comprehension
(7) Oral expression
(8) Written expression

▶ **STROOP COLOR WORLD TEST:**

In the Stroop Color World Test the participant needs to inhibit competing information in order to respond. He will read names of colors printed in different colors, such as the word "red" printed in green. Here vocal and motor speeds are tested and one must make use of working memory to accurately inhibit competing stimuli. Many ADHD individuals find this test challenging.

▶ **WISCONSIN CARD SORTING TEST:**

The Wisconsin Card Sorting Test requires mental flexibility and problem solving ability. Here one must use feedback in his response to formulate the correct pattern based on color, form or number. This test is very useful in evaluating frontal lobe dysfunction in all ADHD cases. These tests are not diagnostic for ADHD and in many cases it is not necessary.

▶ **WHAT ARE THE THREE TYPES OF UNDIAGNOSED ADULT ADHD?**

Generally speaking, we recognize three types of Adult ADHD. In the first group we see adults that act like children with ADHD. Symptoms and actions, responses and impairment of function are quite clear.

In the second group, ADHD symptoms are less obvious. These cases make up the largest group of adult ADHD. They have learned to live with their deficiencies and limitations and to "hide" their condition with coping mechanisms that allow them to function somewhat successfully.

The third group is a small group of adults who deny they have any problem. This group develops rigid compensating mechanisms to keep their lives in order. They live on lists of what to do and where to go. The compensatory methods can be quite complicated. As long as the structure of compensation is working for them, they will function, but the moment one of the lists is lost or an unexpected addition is made, a crisis – big or small –can develop. The inefficient use of time and the endless resources spent on misplaced items or compensating for forgotten appointments or responsibilities as well as the severe limitations as to professional choices take a serious toll. The emotional and financial crises that come from not fully learning from past mistakes and the rigid approach to problem solving also reduces the quality of life. Compensatory behavior often does not extend to social skills.

► **HOW CAN ONE USE THE FULL ASRS?**

One of the most useful scales is the full Adult ADHD Self-Report Scale (ASRS) Symptom Check List VII. This is an 18 item scale that can be used as an initial symptoms assessment to identify adults who might have ADHD. The scale queries adults about the 18 symptoms identified by DSM-IV with modifications to assess adult presentation of ADHD symptoms. The ASRS check list is designed to be a diagnostic aid and is now available through the World Health Organization (WHO).

The following makes up the full Adult Self Rating Scale:
1. Difficulty concentrating when spoken to directly
2. Feeling restless and agitated
3. Trouble wrapping up final details of a project
4. Difficulty unwinding and relaxing during free time
5. Difficulty with tasks requiring organization.
6. Careless mistakes when working on difficult or boring projects
7. Fidgets with hands or feet when sitting for a long period of time
8. Difficulty keeping focus when doing boring or repetitive work
9. Leaves seat when expected to remain in place

Adult ADHD Self Report Score Hyperactivity-Impulsivity:
1. Feeling overactive or compelled to do things
2. Avoiding or delaying tasks that require a lot of thought
3. Talks too much in social situations
4. Misplacing things or has trouble finding belongings
5. Finishing sentences of others
6. Distracted by activities or noise
7. Difficulty waiting
8. Problem remembering appointments or obligations
9. Interrupting others when they are busy.

Each of these symptoms is rated on a frequency basis:

0 – Never
1 – Rarely
2 – Sometimes
3 – Often
4 – Very Often

Once the adult has completed the scale, he can score his result and have a preliminary indication about his self-evaluation. One must keep in mind that the full diagnosis of adult ADHD is dependent on the fulfillment of the three criteria for the diagnosis. Current symptoms will include six inattention and six impulsive-hyperactive symptoms, impairment of function in at least two areas and a history of symptoms during childhood. There are scoring guidelines based on the total score in the inattentive or hyperactive/impulsive subsets that yield a diagnostic likelihood.

► **HOW PREVALENT IS ADULT ADHD IN THE GENERAL POPULATION?**

As reported by many investigators, more than 4% of the adult population experiences significant symptoms of ADHD. The ratio of male to female is about one to one. Most adults with this condition were never diagnosed or treated.

Several studies show that a high percentage of people who were treated for other conditions were found to have untreated ADHD. A national survey of 3200 treated individuals revealed the following findings: Among people who were treated for depression, 13% were also diagnosed as having ADHD that was not treated. Among the people who were treated for anxiety, 9.5% were also diagnosed with ADHD that was not treated. Among those treated for alcohol and drug abuse, 10.8% were also diagnosed with ADHD symptoms. All the respondents experienced ADHD symptoms in the previous 12 months. ADHD is related to an almost three fold increase in the rate of depression and drug abuse in adults.

Since ADHD criteria do not include mood components, many of the overlapping symptoms like distractibility and restlessness seen in depressed adults may mislead the diagnostician.

▶ HOW PREVALENT IS BIPOLAR DISORDER AS AN ASSOCIATED CONDITION IN ADULT ADHD?

Among adults with ADHD, the prevalence of bipolar depression was also three times higher in the national survey conducted in 2006. The most common symptoms in this group was a depressed mood or hopelessness in 33% of the group, mania or hyperactivity in 32%, lack of sleep in 24% and mood swings in 13%.

Another study of depression where patients were followed for 12 years revealed that half were diagnosed with symptoms of depression along with ADHD symptoms. The majority of this group of ADHD adults started to show bipolar symptoms between the ages of 15 and 23.

ADHD ought to be evaluated by an experienced clinician as symptoms of depression may be caused by different factors. Without effective treatment, suicide attempts of this group may reach 45%. Violent episodes and legal problems are much more frequent in this group and as many as 50% may use drugs if not treated. Because of the severity of the symptoms and the impairment of function caused by the combination of the two conditions, a careful diagnosis is critical. Given that about 4% of adults who have ADHD also have bipolar depression, when ADHD adults show mood swings and the symptoms of hyperactivity and impulsivity persist, there is a high likelihood the adult condition may include bipolar depression as well.

▶ IMPORTANT POINTS TO REMEMBER:

- For diagnosis of adult ADHD, six symptoms from the list

of symptoms describing inattention and six symptoms describing impulsive-type behavior need to be present.

- For a diagnosis of adult ADHD, the following conditions need to be fulfilled:

    (1) onset of symptoms prior to age 7

    (2) symptoms cause impairment in two setting such as family and work.

- A self-rating scale is useful in helping each individual assess his condition.

- Among the 4% of adults with ADHD who exhibit these symptoms, a very small percentage are diagnosed and treated effectively.

- Most adults with ADHD have developed mechanisms to compensate for their symptoms or just learned to live with them, although their family and/or work relationships are still often impaired.

Chapter 18

MANAGEMENT OF ADULT ADHD SYMPTOMS

▶ **HOW PREVALENT IS THE TREATMENT OF ADULT ADHD:**

National surveys have shown that only 11% of adults with ADHD received treatment for it in the previous 12 months. That means the vast majority had no treatment intervention at all.

Low ADHD treatment rates were observed even when adults were seen and treated for other psychiatric conditions such as depression, anxiety or alcohol abuse. When primary care physicians were asked about their level of confidence in diagnosing adult ADHD, they reported feeling three times less comfortable diagnosing ADHD than depression. Physicians, as well as the general public, are unclear and sometimes unaware of adult ADHD.

By far, the most effective and consistent way to treat adult ADHD is with medication. Methylphenidate (Ritalin) has been used for more than 50 years for treatment. The results achieved by this medication have been remarkable and consistent. Despite the fact that 70–80% of those taking the medication show improvement, the rate at which this group uses medication remains low. The medical treatment of children, adolescents and adults is identical. The only difference is the dose, adjusted for weight. Once a diagnosis of ADHD is made, adults should implement all the steps discussed earlier from vigorous exercise and balance techniques to Omega 3 and memory exercises

▶ **MUST AN ADULT ACKNOWLEDGE HIS ADHD CONDITION?**

Yes. One of the most important aspects of the treatment of ADHD is to understand its etiology. ADHD *should be regarded as a condition caused by a physical variant in the brain and should be accepted as one would accept diabetes or nearsightedness. It is a chronic condition that will often persist for a lifetime.* It will not improve without intervention.

Although diabetes often persists throughout life, often it can be managed with diet and/or medication. You can also compare it to near-sightedness. Before eyeglasses, near-sightedness might have been considered a real handicap. Today, no one thinks twice about it because it is so easily treated. The neurological deficits underlying ADHD symptoms can be corrected with CPS and BET exercises. Medication can be reduced and finally eliminated as enhanced, quicker and more sophisticated thinking skills develop.

With ADHD, if the symptoms persist into adulthood, only intervention to correct the deficit will be effective. Each symptom and associated condition leads to functional impairment, reduces the quality of life and negatively impacts the potential of most adults with ADHD. *Most are unaware of the degree to which ADHD impinges on their professional and personal lives.*

▶ **HOW CAN UNTREATED ADULT ADHD IMPACT EMPLOYMENT?**

A study of 500 adults who were diagnosed with ADHD as adults indicated that among this group, only 52% were employed. Of the employed adults with ADHD, only 34% were employed on a full time basis, 48% were not currently employed and 14% were actively looking for work.

Among employed ADHD adults who have had more than one job in the past 10 years, 43% report leaving one or more jobs because of ADHD symptoms. For the adult with ADHD, employment history showed that 5.4 different jobs were held during the preceding 10 years as compared to 3.4 jobs held in the same time period by adults without ADHD.

▶ **ARE SOME WORK ENVIRONMENTS BETTER FOR ADHD ADULTS THAN OTHERS?**

Yes. Since impairment in the workplace is such a major problem, adults with ADHD need to evaluate thoroughly which job or profession should be avoided. A good guideline is to capitalize on your strengths. Find work you enjoy and find interesting. Gravitate toward activities that you enjoyed as a young adult and look for diversity in your work. If you have a specific talent or interest, investigate whether this can translate into a business or job. Professions that often accommodate ADHD symptoms include artists, actors, singers, dancers, director, radio/TV positions, video game developers, sports and sports-related activities, independent lawyers, taxi drivers, chefs, tour guides, teachers, marketing and sales.

▶ **ARE THERE WAYS TO PREVENT ADHD SYMPTOMS FROM IMPACTING JOB ADVANCEMENT?**

There are many situations where changes in the work place can make a big difference to the ADHD adult. Many highly successful salesmen find themselves leaving good positions because they do poorly with the required paperwork that must be submitted each week. Discussing your weaknesses with your supervisor and working on a plan for action to solve the problem may lead to greater productivity and a reduction in stress. Talking about your deficit with your boss will allow both of you to address the problem and work on a solution that will make you a better, happier and more productive employee.

Others fail to perform their tasks despite serious efforts on their part to do so. It may be that the tasks can be divided into smaller more manageable parts or communication can be made clearer. Perhaps your supervisor can modify the schedule to reduce the stress. As always, a clear understanding by all of those impacted including supervisors and co-workers can completely change your supervisor's opinion of your performance. You may go from irresponsible and unreliable to motivated and hardworking with a few adjustments. That's a big difference in perception. If an adult with ADHD understands that he will perform better by learning to break long complicated projects into smaller more manageable parts, his performance will be better. Try to minimize distractions by doing difficult tasks early or late in the day when fewer people and activities are taking place.

Another major source of stress and conflict in the workplace for the ADHD adult is social interaction with co-workers and supervisors. Improving social skills is an important goal professionally. Even mild socializing with co-workers will be helpful as far as teamwork and atmosphere in the work place goes.

▶ **HOW SEVERE IS THE IMPACT OF ADULT ADHD SYMPTOMS ON FAMILY AND MARRIAGE?**

The divorce and separation rate for ADHD adults is double the general population. The level of satisfaction in family life was reported to be less than 50% compared with about 70% in non-ADHD adults. Problems include financial difficulties exacerbated by job loss, poor social skills and lack of organization. Parenting conflicts add to the stress.

▶ **WHAT DOES IT TAKE TO KEEP MARRIAGE INTACT?**

For a marriage to be successful, it is imperative that the couple fully understands the etiology of ADHD. For the marriage to continue to grow and develop, both partners must continue to invest time and effort in the relationship. Each needs to feel cared for and loved by the other. The guideline should be: "Accentuate the positive."

Keep in mind your appreciation of your spouse's talents, hard work, and commitment to family. Like other problems, this one can be overcome.

The more common interests and experiences you and your mate share and develop, the closer the relationship will be. Developing common plans and goals will strengthen the bond between you. Real friendship and support should be the ideal goal. When love and equal partnership exist between husband and wife, the partner without ADHD can be an enormous help. As long as there is common respect, love, appreciation and shared goals, helping your spouse to overcome his difficulties can bring additional strength and depth to your relationship.

▶ HOW TO HANDLE STRESS AND CONFLICT IN THE MARRIAGE:

If the relationship is under stress, perhaps the area where dysfunction is highest can be delegated to another person. For example, if finances are a continual source of stress, seek a financial advisor. Adults with ADHD have weak organizational skills and poor attention to details. The goal should be to create financial security and family stability. In the full range of family responsibilities, an ADHD parent may be better at tasks requiring physical activity, such as cooking, yard work, outdoor activities, errands and home maintenance. If one spouse experiences intense frustration in dealing with the children, perhaps responsibilities can be delegated in such a way that the one more emotionally capable of dealing with the children has the lion's share of that responsibility and the other takes over the cooking. Try to be flexible and do what works.

Medication should also be taken as prescribed, especially during stressful times. For reasons which are unclear, a significant number of adults stop taking medication. Optimal progress can be made if the neurotransmitter deficit is corrected. Ideally an adult would use medication until BET is fully implemented.

▶ **CAN AN ADULT WITH ADHD HAVE A SUCCESSFUL MARRIAGE?**

Yes. As in any marriage, success requires commitment, motivation and nurturing. Have a time each week when you review problems as well as progress. Make a list of areas where you are happier and a list of issues you would like to improve. Discuss them in the spirit of enhancing your life together. Keep in mind that you will not solve all problems quickly or all at one time. Every time you successfully resolve an issue, you will be able to take that experience and apply it to new situations. If you have continuing difficulties in any of these areas, do not hesitate to seek professional help. With proper intervention a couple can learn to handle more complicated issues between them over time. There are few relationships in life more important than that between husband and wife. Do not give up. Work diligently to find solutions and accentuate the positive emotions between you.

▶ **DO ADHD SYMPTOMS IMPACT SEXUAL RELATIONSHIPS?**

There are some reports of highly energetic people that become so involved in so many activities that by the time they go to bed, they lose interest in sex. Since they put all their energy into their activities during the day, they have little energy left by the end of the day. The spouse should not take this as a personal rejection. They should instead gently guide their partner in the right direction. Others may need sexual stimulation so often that the spouse is exhausted. This issue is easy to resolve as long as the underlying relationship is good and these issues are discussed in a light and seductive way. One should also keep in mind that poor social skills can carry over into the sexual relationship and again, this doesn't mean the person is cold or insensitive or unloving. Keep this in mind and respond in a loving way.

▶ **HOW CAN PARENTAL ISSUES BE HANDLED EFFECTIVELY?**

One of the more complicated issues involves parenting. Adult ADHD symptoms can cause constant difficulties in parenting especially if the child also has ADHD. Inconsistent behavior exhibited by most ADHD adults as well as low frustration tolerance adds to the stress of raising children.

The most critical step for all adults with ADHD is to develop a common agreement with their spouse on all issues related to parenting. This cannot be over-emphasized.

▶ **CAN MARRIAGE ADAPT TO ADHD IN THE RELATIONSHIP?**

To have problems managed more effectively in the marriage, tasks and responsibilities should be discussed. A special notebook or bulletin board should be used to keep track of household responsibilities and tasks. Review this on a regular basis and act accordingly. These personal tasks, when consistently performed, will help sustain and enhance the marriage. When husband and wife are friends and partners in life, then ADHD is dealt with as one of life's challenges. Sharing feelings, wishes, needs and disappointments openly will give a couple the strength they need to meet challenges and grow the love between them with open communication and trust.

Having to "check off" tasks as they are completed helps to prevent procrastination and forgetfulness.

Never forget gratitude.

► CAN SOCIAL SKILLS BE IMPROVED?

Many adults with ADHD exhibit serious deficits when it comes to relationships, socialization and the ability to sustain friendships or make new friends. Their poor social skills can be manifested by impulsive comments, short temper, verbal abuse and failure to appreciate other's needs. Their poor listening may make them appear immature. *Unfortunately, most adults with* ADHD *do not recognize their serious social deficits.* The good news is that most of these skills can be coached, practiced and mastered.

The key to learning new social skills is first to recognize that they are lacking. Most successful Olympic champions watch their performance in practice or in actual competition again and again so that they can identify their weaknesses in order to correct them. Adults with ADHD have to adopt the same strategy and recognize their specific areas of weakness and work diligently to improve these lagging skills.

Focus your first effort on improving your listening skills. This is the most valuable trait you can develop. Everyone appreciates a good listener. It is a critical asset anyone can master. Express interest by body language, facial expression and empathy. A number of adults have reported using the "technique" of biting softly on the inside of their cheek to remind themselves to stay focused and listen. Once you have mastered the art of listening, you can concentrate on the next social skill that needs to be improved. You are not going to be an expert immediately any more than you can play an excellent game of tennis the first time you pick up a racket. Do not give up; you can be successful. Anger and impulsive inappropriate comments will be much easier to control if your goal is to be the best listener in the room.

► CAN YOU LEARN TO IDENTIFY "TRIGGERS" THAT LEAD TO MALADAPTIVE SOCIAL RESPONSES?

There are several common triggers that result in a negative overreaction. When you try to work on these social skills, you must identify many of the triggers that cause you to lose control. Once you have identified these, memorize them.

These stimuli may be the only warning signal you receive before you lose control. Teach yourself a more productive way to express your frustration and anger. Controlling anger is not a simple task, and keep in mind that the longer you have been using maladaptive responses, the longer it will take to correct the behavior.

▶ **CAN RELATIONSHIPS BE ENHANCED AND IMPROVED WITH NEW SOCIAL SKILLS?**

Making new friends and sustaining friendships will become easier once social skills improve. To sustain friendships, you need to review the attributes you appreciate in your friend and the interests you have in common. Be proactive; include friends in common activities. Stay in touch. Develop a social calendar where you initiate group activities. Relaxed social activities such as dinner out with another couple or going to the theater are good places to begin. In the beginning, think of activities such as movies or musical entertainment where you can enjoy activities together, but do not feel pressure to converse extensively. Your social skills will improve and gradually friendship will develop.

▶ **IMPORTANT POINTS TO REMEMBER:**
- Commit yourself to daily mental and physical exercise. Refer to Brain Exercise Therapy.
- The first and most important aspect of ADHD treatment is to understand the etiology of the condition and accept it and its symptoms.
- To minimize functional impairment in the work place, one needs to capitalize on personal strengths, interests, work diversity and personal preferences in choosing a career.
- An aptitude test may help bring into focus specific strengths and abilities.

- It is important to find areas where you can excel and that you find interesting.
- Many conflicts at work can be reduced by discussing how you can work optimally with your supervisor.
- Dividing work tasks into smaller more manageable parts will improve work performance.
- Using an outside advisor to deal with financial management may significantly reduce family stress.
- Investing time and effort in the marital relationship will help create a common ground for rules in raising the children and in facing life's many challenges.
- Sexual issues have a solution.
- Develop common interests and social activities to enhance marital bonds and strengthen the relationship.
- Try to define family responsibilities in terms of each person's strengths.
- An ADHD adult will contribute more to the marriage by taking on responsibilities that emphasize capabilities rather than weaknesses.
- Find an expert to assume responsibility when a particular activity is a weak point for both partners.
- Always work to open communication and limit criticism.
- Social skills can be improved by learning to listen and controlling impulsive comments.
- Ask your wife/husband or close friend or relative to point out specific social weaknesses so that you can work on overcoming them.
- Identify triggers that cause you to overreact in specific situations. Memorize these stimuli and use them as warning signals to develop better self-control.
- When you get up in the morning and before you go to bed at night, recite a list of the good things in your life. Do it every day. Try it while brushing your teeth.

Chapter 19

MEDICAL TREATMENT OF ADHD

► **BENEFITS AND LIMITATIONS OF RITALIN**

If your child needed to wear corrective shoes, you wouldn't hesitate to get them. While you wouldn't continue with the corrective shoes after successful treatment, it would be foolish to only wear them for a few weeks and then conclude that they don't help. When Ritalin doesn't seem to be working, both professionals and parents sometimes take the child off the drug before confirming the dose is sufficient. Ritalin is only the beginning. The goal is to improve brain function to the point where Ritalin is no longer necessary. However it is much easier to accomplish this when working with a child whose symptoms are minimal. Ritalin is effective in about 70% of ADHD cases. If the dose is right, and Ritalin still does not relieve ADHD symptoms, another treatment should be implemented.

► **IS RITALIN (METHYLPHENIDATE) EFFECTIVE IN THE TREATMENT OF ADHD?**

Yes. ADHD is by far the most commonly diagnosed neurobehavioral condition in children and continues to impact individuals

throughout the life cycle. One should consider several pharma-
cological agents in the treatment of ADHD. Significant evidence
supports the role of certain medications as a critical part of treatment.

Over one hundred controlled studies with more than 5000
children and adolescents have documented the efficacy of medication in about 70% of patients. Stimulants are the first line of
therapy and are among the most well studied and most established treatment for ADHD. The literature clearly supports that
methylphenidate not only improve behavior, but also self-esteem,
cognition, and general functioning by enhancing mental focus
and behavior. This class of drugs diminishes the symptoms of inattention, hyperactivity and impulsivity. The use of methylphenidate can help performance in school as well. There is more positive feedback from school, less conflict at home and improved
peer relationships. Of course, a diagnosis of ADHD coupled
with a complete medical examination to rule out such things as
congenital heart abnormalities is necessary before starting any
medication. The most commonly used medications for ADHD are
Ritalin and Aderall as well as the long-acting equivalent medication, Concerta, Ritalin LA and Aderall XR. Just keep in mind that
Ritalin only temporarily corrects the neurotransmitter deficiency.
The goal is to eliminate the need for medication.

▶ **DO WE UNDERSTAND HOW RITALIN WORKS?**

Yes. One of the most essential neurotransmitters in the brain is
dopamine. Dopamine is found in the mid-brain and it's function
is transmitting messages to the prefrontal areas of the brain. This
is similar to an electrical signal traveling from one point to another. If, for any reason, there is a deficit of dopamine, this signal
is dramatically weakened. At each neuronal synapse, dopamine
is released and in normal circumstances, diffuses across a microscopic space to lock on to a receptor on the surface of the next

neuron. Contact with the receptor triggers a conduction impulse. A transporter molecule in the synaptic space acts to recycle dopamine once its job is done, carrying it back to its storage site for re-use. *If the body produces too many transporter molecules at the synapse, much of the dopamine never reaches its intended receptor sites.* The resulting signal is weak and is expressed as impulsivity (because the inhibitory signal is weak) or a lack of concentration and agitation (because the stimulatory signal is weak).

This is the point where stimulants such as methylphenidate come into play. An individual with ADHD produces too many transporter molecules. Ritalin ties up the excess transporter molecules so that all the dopamine molecules reach their intended receptor site and function normally. Ritalin reaches the brain after about 15 minutes when taken orally, with the medication reaching peak effect in about 2 hours. If taken at 7:30 in the morning, the peek effect will be at about 9:30 A.M. By 11:30 in the morning, about 4 hours after administering the medication, most of the benefits of the medication have subsided and Ritalin is no longer in circulation.

▶ **IS RITALIN ADDICTIVE?**

No. The chemical structure of Ritalin is similar to that of cocaine, and this has led of concerns about addiction. Methylpenidate (Ritalin) is not addictive. Both cocaine and Ritalin can cause an increase in dopamine concentration at the neuronal synapse. However, the rate of initial uptake and eventual clearance from the brain of these two chemicals is drastically different. Injected cocaine starts to impact the brain within 5–8 seconds and reaches peak effect in about 4 minutes, while orally ingested Ritalin only starts to reach the brain within 15 minutes, with peak effect taking place after 2 hours and clearance from the system concluding around 4 hours after taking the medication.

The initial fast uptake of cocaine into the brain is responsible for the "high" experienced by drug addicts. The slow release of Ritalin from the brain cells interferes with frequent repeat administration and lessens its addictive potential, whereas cocaine is highly addictive. Any medication, even aspirin, can be abused. However, for Ritalin to be abused, a person would have to take many pills at once and even then, the effect would be quite mild compared to injected cocaine.

▶ **WHAT IS THE MOST EFFECTIVE WAY TO USE RITALIN?**

It is best to start with a low dose of Ritalin and gradually increase it to optimal benefit. The guideline that seems most effective and helps the body adjust to the new medication is to start with a dose of 0.3mg for each kilogram of body weight per day for children or adults. The FDA has approved up to 60 mg per day reflecting an optimal level of about 1 mg for each kilogram of body weight per day. This level can be reached by gradually increasing the dosage during the first three weeks of treatment. Studies have shown that improvement in functioning and remission of symptoms were related to the dosage level of medication administered. One must remember that to correct a neurological deficit and achieve optimal neuronal functioning, the dose must be correct. The higher the dose, the greater the proportion of children who achieved full benefit. It is vital to be aware that with all drugs, even aspirin, one can overdose and therefore, careful monitoring in the first stage of treatment is necessary to achieve safe and optimal results.

As one observes and monitors each of the symptoms, one should rate the behavioral changes for each symptom out of the 18 DSM IV symptom list:
- Symptoms not present at all
- infrequently present
- frequently present
- present most of the time

If parents and teachers carefully score and monitor the child on a weekly basis, an accurate reflection of the effects of the medication can be determined.

▶ **IS LONG-ACTING RITALIN MORE EFFECTIVE IN TREATMENT?**

A new form of methylpenidate was developed in the last few years that has markedly changed the treatment of ADHD. This long-acting agent has extended release for up to 12 hours.

Concerta (long-acting methylpenidate) allows the gradual release from a capsule and doesn't require taking medication three times a day. The capsule is designed to release the medication in such a way as to maintain a constant level of methylphenidate for 12 hours. "Ritalin LA" is another long acting agent with an 8 hour duration in a constant level of methylphenidate is maintained. With these daily doses, a substantially higher recovery rate and higher rate of compliance can be achieved. Parents no longer need to administer medication three times a day or worry about getting the medication to school.

Because compliance is better and the long acting agents seem to get a smoother response from children throughout the day, symptom management is better. Another important advantage in using long acting agents is the fact that extended release stimulants are rarely abused.

▶ **WHAT ARE THE SIDE EFFECTS ASSOCIATED WITH RITALIN?**

The most commonly reported side effects associated with methylphenidate are appetite suppression and sleep problems. There have been some reports of mood disturbance ranging from increased tearfulness to major depression, but it's not clear in these cases if there was an underlying psychological difficulty beforehand.

Rarely, side effects include high blood pressure, increased heart rate, vomiting and nausea.

Other infrequent side effects include headaches, restlessness, abdominal discomfort and occasionally fatigue or depression. No known damage has been associated with the medically supervised use of Ritalin, which has been used for the last 40 years according to medical literature with only a small percentage reporting side effects. I am recommending that if medication is necessary according to medical evaluation, you should view it as temporary. The goal is to eliminate the need for medication.

▶ **WHAT ARE THE NEW GUIDELINES RECOMMENDED BY THE FDA?**

The FDA's guidelines are intended for those with potential cardiovascular and psychiatric risks. They report Ritalin risks for children, adolescents and adults with *structural* cardiac abnormalities or other serious heart conditions. For adults, the use of ADHD drugs are not recommended for those with structural cardiac abnormalities, serious heart rhythm abnormalities, coronary disease or other heart problems. It is important to monitor blood pressure and heart rate before beginning treatment. Patients with preexisting psychiatric illness, family history of suicide, bipolar illness or depression, need to be aware that taking stimulant medication may exacerbate symptoms of behavior disturbance and thought disorders.

Clear answers about the potential stunting of height and weight with the use of stimulants has yet to be found unless used for years. The latest study in 2007 indicate that after constant use for 2 years there was a small reduction in height reported but within a few years after the drug was discontinued, the full growth expected for the child returns. Not enough studies have been done to be definitive. Ideally Ritalin would only be used in the initial stages of treatment until strategies such as CPS and BET improve brain function which should average about three to six months.

All medication has side effects but so does having no

treatment at all. Symptoms resulting from no treatment can be poor self esteem, low confidence, dismal academic performance, risky behavior, impulsivity, career limitations, etc.

▶ **WHAT IS THE MOST EFFECTIVE WAY TO DEAL WITH THE SIDE EFFECTS OF RITALIN?**

The most common side effect is loss of appetite, so weight loss needs to be monitored on a weekly basis. Usually weight stabilizes and parents should try to give the medication with food, add calorie-rich healthy snacks, and serve food the child likes. For children who are extremely picky eaters, you might want to take a look at cook books such as "The Sneaky Chef" and "Deceptively Delicious" which enhances the nutritional value of kid friendly food. Sleep problems can often be managed by lowering the dose in the afternoon. Paradoxically, increasing the dose can sometimes be useful as it helps the child to organize himself better for sleep. Doing obvious things like avoiding exciting activities right before bedtime and maintaining a calm routine are helpful. Participating in a quiet activity about 30 minutes before bedtime as well as avoiding any TV or other noisy activity can help the child fall asleep more easily. Using a long acting agent will cut down on the 'rebound' phenomenon seen when the four hour effect of regular Ritalin is over. When medication is cleared from the system, the condition of too many transporter molecules returns. If the child is upset or agitated about something at home or school, this will be reflected in restlessness, an inability to sleep or emotional outbursts. Always investigate what happened to your child at school when you see these symptoms. Perhaps he had a fight with a friend or feels insecure. Keep in mind that unlike antibiotics, one can stop taking Ritalin at any time and it will be clear the body within hours.

Are there other medications besides Ritalin that can be used?

Yes. Aderall, like Ritalin, is a stimulant that has a similar effect on neurotransmitters. Aderall XR is the long acting equivalent which lasts 12 hours. Both Aderall and Ritalin produce similar positive results. For some, one works better than the other, but Ritalin has less abuse potential.

Are there non-stimulant medications to treat ADHD?

Yes. Strattera (atamoxatine) is a relatively new medication that was approved by the FDA in 2003 to be used exclusively for the treatment of adult ADHD. Strattera improves neural conduction by inhibiting the uptake of norepinephrine at the synapse, which increases the concentration of neurotransmitters and the strength of impulse conduction. Strattera has a completely different molecular structure and is not related to stimulants. To reach an optimal effect with Strattera, one needs to take it much longer to see results. Optimal results are usually achieved by giving one to one and a half mg per kg of body weight per day. However, one must start with a lower dose and gradually increase to an optimal level. It may take three to four weeks to reach this optimal level, whereas with Ritalin optimal results can be reached within two hours. The side effects of Strattera which are rare include nausea, vomiting, dry mouth, and sedation. In some cases, urinary retention and erectile dysfunction have been noted. It has also been linked to suicidal thoughts.

Can anti-depressant medication be used to treat ADHD?

Yes. Tri-cyclic anti-depressants such as desipramine and amitryptyline that were originally used to treat depression, have been used successfully to treat ADHD as well. The use of a very low dose of desipramine (10mg/day) may relieve some ADHD symptoms with few side effects. Some of the side effects reported include skin eruptions, constipation, urinary retention, dry mouth and drowsiness. The most serious side effect of this type of medication is heart arrhythmias. This is a serious medical complication that requires ECG monitoring during treatment.

Are there other medications that can be used?

Yes. Bupropion, commericially known as Zyban and Wellbutrin can be used as an alternative but often produces poor results. Bupropion is not as effective as Ritalin but in some cases, the results are surprisingly good. It may also be useful in treating people who wish to stop smoking. Side effects may include anxiety, insomnia and rarely, seizures. In rare cases, some medication to treat high blood pressure can be used to treat ADHD.

▶ **HOW EFFECTIVE IS MEDICAL TREATMENT?**

Hundreds of well-controlled studies document the safety and efficacy of treating children and adults with ADHD. Methylphenidate has been shown to provide the greatest efficacy. A review of 15 different ADHD medications and studies on nearly 11,500 patients indicated that methylphenidate-like medication exhibited greater effect compared with non-stimulant medications.

Adherence rates tend to be better with the newer extended release capsules. Only once parents and patients fully understand the benefits of medication in the treatment of ADHD will adherence rates increase. Poor usage rates are compounded by bad press and unfounded fears associated with medicating children. True, there are side effects and medical monitoring is necessary. However, most would agree that the benefits far outweigh the liabilities. Without treatment, there is a relentless daily assault on self-esteem and confidence that can have a permanent effect on personality and character. In addition, untreated ADHD can be a danger as illustrated by the dramatic increase in accidents and risky behavior. The good news is that applying the methods and strategies discussed in this book can reduce the need for medication or eliminate it altogether. That is the ultimate goal. Medication is often useful in the early stages of treatment.

▶ **IMPORTANT POINTS TO REMEMBER:**

- The medications that treat ADHD have been used for over

70 years. They are well-studied and have been established as first line of therapy.

- Hundreds of controlled studies document the safety and efficacy of treatment in both children and adults.
- Methylphenidate increases the level of dopamine in the brains of ADHD individuals who have low levels of this neurotransmitter.
- Although the chemical structure of cocaine and methylphenidate are similar, methylphenidate is not addictive when taken as prescribed. To abuse methylphenidate, it would have to be taken in huge quantities.
- Using long acting methylphenidate gives a smoother, more consistent response that lasts for 12 hours.
- Long acting methylphenidate is very rarely abused.
- The most common side effects of methylphenidate are appetite suppression and sometimes sleep problems.
- There are potential cardiovascular and psychiatric risks associated with the use of ADHD medication by those with a history of structural cardiac abnormalities, pre-existing psychiatric conditions, or family history of psychiatric problems.
- Amphetamine-type medications seem to be quite effective for treatment, but do have significant potential for abuse and may impact the cardiovascular system.
- Atomoxetine, Imipramine. and Buprofin are medications that also can be used as a second line of treatment in cases where methylphenidate is not effective.
- The use of medication in the treatment of ADHD can be reduced and often eliminated by using the strategies discussed in this book.

Chapter 20

CONCLUSION

This book has been a family affair with contributions from my wife and daughter-in-law. They have enriched this book with their areas of expertise as well as their personal and professional experience with ADHD. If you would like to be in touch with questions or comments, I will answer as soon as possible. Web site: www.tocureADHD.com

I have summarized the most recent findings concerning ADHD from the most prestigious research facilities in the world. In addition to my own professional experiences, I have relied on treatment results with children, teenagers and adults across a broad spectrum of those involved in professional practice and those involved in academic research. The conclusions are difficult to dispute: BET and CPS combined with unconditional emotional support and utilization of all the strategies appropriate for your child can lead to success. The most dramatic results absolutely require implementing all aspects of treatment. Professionals like myself can aid in training, help with difficult problems, give advice, answer questions, provide guidance and make sure you get a good start. Do not hesitate to use professional resources.

However, this book is designed for you, the parents. You can be a great parent-coach for your child. As an added benefit, it may bring your family closer together.

You will develop skills and confidence in your ability to coach your child and be able to give him direction and guidance while encouraging independence and self reliance.

You have every reason to be positive, optimistic, and motivated about bringing out the best in your child and helping him be all that he can be. There is no better time to start than right now.

When you analyze all the components of BET and CPS plus all the other strategies, you will notice that the expense involved is minimal. Structuring conversations to be learning experiences through CPS and MLE, using praise and rewards for jobs well done, building your child's confidence and self esteem cost nothing at all and have powerful results. The most comforting aspect of this approach is that it is totally natural and the body's own potential corrects deficiencies. Medication may help in the beginning but the goal is to eliminate all drugs. Since ADHD is a real biological condition, you will need to keep regular visits with your doctor for follow-up. Bring your notebook to go over all the successes and problems and make sure you are getting the maximum benefit from your efforts. Adults who have never been treated for ADHD symptoms may need professional assistance, but the goal is for the therapist to gradually work his way out of a job.

This is a time of great discovery and possibilities. Even as this book is ready to be published, more of the mysteries of ADHD succumb to scientific research and our understanding increases exponentially. From the 54th Annual Meeting of the American Academy of Child and Adolescent Psychiatry 2007, magnetic resonance imaging (MRI) studies show that adults with ADHD have smaller cortical areas and volume deficits exactly where attention and executive functions are located. Most of the subjects had a relatively high IQ and most were college educated. Altering mental habits, learning new information, adapting to different more sophisticated patterns and creating new memories enhance brain growth and development. Our brains can generate new cells and possess a lifelong ability to absorb new memories and learn new skills. ADHD is a challenge to be confronted and cured. Every step along the way brings with it a sense of accomplishment and success. It is wonderful that the best, most effective treatment is healthy, has no unpleasant side effects and promotes brain growth.

Remember, Ritalin does nothing to directly influence emotional regulation and immaturity nor to improve language, thinking or social skills.

Be pro-active, feel good about yourself, and know that success is around the corner.

If you want to contact me with questions or comments, please go to: www.tocureADHD.com. I will answer all emails as soon as possible.

References:

Introduction

1) Biederman J., Spencer T. Attention-deficit/hyperactivity disorder (ADHD) as noradrenergic disorder. Biol. Psychitry 1999:46:1234–42.

2) Jensen PS, Hinshaw SP, Swanson JM, et.al. Finding from the NIMH Multimodel Treatment Study of ADHD (MTA) implications and pplictions for primary care providers. J. Dev. Behav. Pediatr. 2001: 22:60–73.

3) Stevens J., Quittner A.L., Abikoff H. (1998) Factors influencing elementary school teachers' ratings of ADHD and ADD behaviours. Journal of Clinical Child Psychology 27(4), 406–414.

4) A 14 month randomized clinical trial of treatment strategies for attention deficit hyperactivity disorder. The MTA cooperative Group. Multimodel Treatment Study of Children with ADHD. Arch. Gen. Psychiatry. 1999:56: 1073–1086.

5) Conners, CK Forty years of methylphenidate treatment in Attention-Deficit Hyperactivity Disorder. J. Atten. Disorder 2002: 6 (suppl): 517–530.

6) Luria, A.R. Higher Cortical Functions in Man. 1966. Basic Books. New York, NY.

Chapter 1

1) Faraone SV, Beiderman J, Krifcher Lehman B, et.al. Intellectual performance and school failure in children with attention deficit hyper-

activitydisorder and in their siblings. J. Abnormal Psychol. 1993: 102: 616–623.

2) Brown, T.E., Attention-Deficit Disorder and CoMorbidities in children, adolescents and adults. 1st Ed. Arlington, Va. American Psychiatric Publishing, Inc.: 2000.

3) Beiderman, et.al A controlled study of functional impairments. J. Clin. Psychiatry 2006:67:524.

Chapter 2

1) American Psychiatric Association (1994) Diagnostic and statistical manual of mental disorders (4th ed) Washington, D.C.

2) Brooker BH, Cyr JJ: Tables for clinicians to use to convert WAIS-R short Forms. Journal Clinical Psychology 1986: 42: 983–986.

3) Doyle AE, Biederman J, Seidman LJ, Weber W, Faraone SV. Diagnostic Efficiency of neuropsychological test scores for discriminating boys with and without ADHD. Journal of Consulting Clinical Psychology 2000: 68: 477–488.

4) Golden CJ: Stroop Color and Word Test. A manual for clinical and experimental use. Chicago, Stoelting Co. 1978.

5) Heaton RK, Chelune GJ, Talley JL, et.al. Wisconsin Card Sorting Test Manual: Revised and expanding. Odessa, Fl. Psychological Assessment Resources Inc. 1993.

Chapter 3

1) Bush G., Frazier, JA, Rauch SL, Siedman LJ, Whalen PJ, Jenike MA, Rosen BR, Biederman J. Anterior cingulate cortex dysfunction in Attention Deficit Hyperactivity Disorder revealing by FMRI and the Counting Stroop. Biological Psychiatry 1999: 45: 1542–1552.

2) Zanetkin AJ, Nordahl TE, Gross M, et.al. Cerebral glucose metabolism in In adults with hyperactivity in childhood onset. New England Journal of Medicine 1990: 323: 1361–1366.

3) Castellonose F, Giedd J, Marsh W, Hamburger S, et.al. (1996) Quantitative brain magnetic resonance imaging in attention deficit hyperactivity disorder.

4) Bush et.al. 2003. Modified from Bush, Luu and Posner. Trends in Cognitive Sciences 2000: 4; 215–222.

5) Valera E, Faraone SV, Biederman J, et.al. Functional neuroanatomy of Working memory in adults with ADHD. Biological Psychiatry 2005.

6) Volkow ND, Wang G, Fowler JS, et.al. (2001) Therapeutic doses of oral methylphenidate significantly increases extracellular dopamine in the human brain. J. Neurosci. 21, RC (2).

7) Bush G, Frazier JA, Rauch SL, et.al. Anterior cingulated cortex Dysfunction in attention deficit hyperactivity disorder revealed by FMRI and the Counting Stroop. Biological Psychiatry 1999: 45: 1542–1552.

8) Faraone SV, Khan SA. Candidate gene studies of attention deficit Hyperactivity disorder. J. Clin. Psychiatry 2006: 67; 13–20.

Chapter 4

1) Spenser T, Biederman J, Wilens T. Attention deficit hyperactivity disorder . and comorbidity. Pediatr. Clin. North Am. 46 (5): 915–927, Oct 1999.

2) Kurlan, McDermoth, Deeley, et al. Prevalence of Tics in school children and association with placement in special education. Neurology 2001: 57, 1383–1388.

3) Semrud-Clikeman MS, Biederman J, Sprich S, et.al. Comorbidity between ADHD and learning disabilities: A review and report in a clinically referred sample. J Am Acad Child. Adolesc. Psychiatry 1992: 31: 439–443.

4) Biderman J, Faraone S, Spencer T, et.al. Growth deficits and ADHD Revisited: Impact of gender, development and treatment.

5) Faraone SV, Biederman J, Mennim D, et.al. Attention-deficit hyperactivity disorder with bipolar disorder: a familial subtype. J Am Acad Child Adolesc Psychiatry 1997: 36(10): 1378–87.

6) Faraone SV, Doyle AE. The nature and heritability of attention deficit Hyperactivity disorder. Child Adolesc Psychiatry Clin N Am. 2001: 10 (2): 299–316.

7) Mill J, Curran S, Richards S, Taylor E, Asherson P. Polymorphisms in the Dopamine D5 receptor (DRDS) Gene and ADHD. Am J Med Genet 13 Neuropsychiatr Gend 125 (1): 38–42, Feb 2004.

8) Farone SV, Biderman J, Weiffenbach B. Dopamine D4 Gene 7- Repeat Allele and attention deficit hyperactivity disorder. Am J Psychiatry 156 (5): 768–770, 1999.

9) Ponerleau O, Downey K, Stelson F, Pomerleau O. (1995) Cigarette smoking in adult patients diagnosed with attention deficit hyperactivity disorder. Journal of Substance Abuse 7:L 373–378.

10) Milberger S, Biederman J, Faraone S, et.al. Is maternal smoking during pregnancy a risk factor for attention deficit hyperactivity disorder in children? Am J Psychiatry 153: 1138–1142.

11) Biederman J, Farone SV, Mick E, et.al High risk for attention deficit Hyperactivity disorder among children of parents with childhood onset of the disorder: Am J Psychiatry 1995. 152: 431–435.

12) Castellanos F, Lee P, et.al. Developmental trajectories of brain volume abnormalities in children and adolescents with ADHD (2002) JAMA 288: 1740–1748.

13) Hallowell EM and Ratey JJ. Delivered from Distraction. 2006. Ballentine Books: New York. 177–1186

13) Hallowell EM and Ratey JJ. Delivered from Distraction. 2006. Ballentine Books: New York. 177–1186.

Chapter 5

1) Hodgkins P, Boken M, Capone NM, et.al. Office visits and prescriptionfill rates in patients with ADHD. Program and abstracts of the 19th U.S. Psychiatric and Mental Health Congress: Nov. 15–19, 2006. New Orleans, La.

2) Barkley, RA (1997). Defiant children: A clinician's manual for parent training. New York: Guilford Press.

3) Baumrind D (1968). Authoritarian vs authoritative parent control. Adolescence 3: 255–272.

4) Faraone SV, Biederman J, Kiely K. Cognitive functioning, learning disability and school failure in attention deficit hyperactivity disorder. Edited by Beitchman J. Essex, England. Cambridge University Press 1996.

5) Seidman LJ, Biederman J, Faraone S, et.al. Effects of family history and Comorbidity on the neuropsychological performance of ADHD children. J Am Acad Child Adolesc Psychiatry 1995: 34; 1015–1024.

6) Beiderman J, Faraone SV, Keenan K, et.al. Family-genetic and Psychosocial risk factors in DSM III attention deficit disorder. J Am Acad Child Adolesc Psychiatry 1990: 29; 526–533.

7) Minuchin S. 1974: Families and family therapy. Cambridge, Ma. Harvard University Press.

Chapter 6

1) Kazdin AE, (1997). Parent management trainingt: Evidence, outcome

and issues. Journal of the American Academy of Child and Adolescent Psychiatry, 36 (10) 1349–1356.

2) Proffer AA (1996) The interpersonal treatment of young children: Principles and techniques. Psychotherapy 33 (1) 68–76.

3) Douglas VI. Stop, Look and Listen: The problem of sustained attention and impulse control in hyperactive and normal children. Canadian J of Behavioral Science 1972. 4: 259–282.

4) Belsky J (1984) The determination of parenting: A process model. Child Development 55: 83–96.

5) Bernal ME, Klinner MD, Schultz LA. (1980) Outcome evaluation of behavioural parent training and client-centered parent counselling for children with conduct problem. J of Applied Behavior Analysis 13: 677–691.

6) Cavell TA (2000) Working with parents of aggressive children. Washington D.C. American Psychological Assoc.

7) Chamberlin P, Patterson GR (1995) Discipline and child compliance in Parenting. In MH Bornstein (Ed) Handbook of parenting Vol 4. Applied and practical parenting. 205–225. Mahwah NJ: Erlbaum.

8) Dumas JE and La Freniere PJ (1993) Mother-Child relationships as sources of support or stress. A comparison of competent average and aggressive and anxious days. Child Development 64: 1732–1754.

9) Gerard AB (1994). Parent-child relationship inventory (PCR1) Los Angeles: Western Psychological Services.

10) Kazdin AE (1997) Parent management training: Evidence, outcome and issues. J American Academy of Child and Adolescent Psychiatry 36 (10) 1349–1356.

Chapter 7

1) Gardner, FM. 1989. Inconsistent parenting: Is there evidence for a link with children's conduct problems? J of Abnormal Child Psychology 17: 223–233.

2) Biderman J, Menuteus MC, Doyle AE, et.al. Impact of executive function Deficits and attention deficit hyperactivity disorder on academic outcomes in children. J of Consulting and Clinical Psychology 72: 757–766. 2004.

3) Anastopoules AD, Guevremont D, Shelton TL, et.al. (1992) Parenting Stress among families with attention deficit hyperactivity disorder. J of Abnormal Child Psychology 20: 503–520.

Chapter 8

1) Goldman LS, Genel M, Bezman RJ, et.al. Diagnosis and treatment of Attention deficit/hyperactivity disorder in children and adolescents. JAMA 1998: 279: 1100–1107.

2) Alexander JF, Parsens BV (1973). Behavioral family interventions with delinquent families. Impact on family process and recidivism. J of Abnormal Psychology 81: 219–225.

3) Taylor TK and Biglan A. (1998) Behavioral family interventions for improving child rearing. A review of the literature for clinician and policy makers. Clinical Child and Family Review 1 (1) 41–60.

Chapter 9

1) Greene RW. The Explosive Child (2001). A new approach for understanding and parenting easily frustrated chronically inflexible children. New York: Harper Collins.

2) Kendall PC (1993) Cognitive-behavioral therapies with youth: Guiding theory, current status and emerging developments. J of Consulting and Clinical Psychology 61: (2) 235–247.

3) Brestan EV and Eybeg SM. (1998) Effective psychological treatment of Conduct disordered children and adolescents. 29 years, 82 studies and 5,272 kids. J of Clinical Child Psychology 27 (2) 180–189.

4) Gardner FM (1989) Inconsistent parenting: Is there evidence for a link With children's conduct problems. J of Abnormal Child Psychology 17: 223–233.

5) Bloomquist ML, August GJ, Cohen C, et.al. Social problem solving in Hyperactive-aggressive children: How and what they think in conditions of controlled processing. J of Clinical Child Psychology 26: 172–180

6) Pennington BF and Ozonoff S. (1996) Executive functions and Developmental psychopathology. J of Child Psychology and Psychiatry 37: 51–87.

7) Kendall PC (1993) Cognitive-behavioral therapies with youth: Guiding Theory current status and emerging development. J of Consulting and Clinical Psychology 61 (2): 235–247.

Chapter 10

1) Greene, RW and Ablou SA (2006) Treating explosive kids: The Collaborative Problem Solving Approach. New York: Guilford Press.

2) Greene RW, Ablon SA and Goring JC. (2003) A transactional model of Oppositional behaviour. Underpinning of the Collaborative Problem Solving Approach. J of Psychosomatic Research 55: 67–75.

3) Greene RW, Ablon JS, Monuteaux M, et.al. (2001) Effectiveness of Collaborative problem solving in affectively dysregulated youth with oppositional defiant disorder: J of Consulting and Clinical Psychology 72 (6) 1157–1164.

4) Kazdin AE, Siegel TC and Bass D (1992) Cognitive problem solving skills Training and parent management in the treatment of antisocial behaviour in children. J of Consulting and Clinical Psychology 60 (5) 733–747.

Chapter 11

1) Bavelier D and Neville H. 2002 Neuroplasticisty developmental. In V.S. Ramachandran Ed. Academic Press, 561.

2) Rosenzweig D, Krech EL, Bennet MC, et.al. 1962. Effects of Environmental complexity and training on chemistry and anatomy: J of Comparative and Physiological Psychology 55: 429–37.

3) Turner AM and Greenough WT. 1985. Differential rearing effectis on rat visual cortex synapses. Synaptic and neuronal density and synapses per neuron. Brain Research 329: 195–203.

4) Rosenzweig, MR. 1996. Aspects of the search for neural mechanisms of memory. Annual Review of Psychology 47: 1–32.

5) Merzenich MM, Tallal P, Petersen S, et.al. (1999) Neuronal plasticity: Building a bridge from the laboratory to the clinic. Berlin: Springer-Verlag, 169–87.

6) Edelman GM and Tonomi G. 2000. A Universe of Consciousness. New York Basic Books, 38.

7) Temple, GK, Deutsch, RA, Poldrack, SL, et.al. 2003. Neural deficits in Children with dyslexia ameliorated by behavioural remediation: Evidence from functional MRI. Proceedings of the National Academy of Sciences, U.S.A. 100 (5) 2860–65.

8) Nagarajan DT, Blake DT, Wright BA, et.al. 1998. Practice-related improvements in somatosensory interval discrimination are temporally specific but generalized across skill location, hemisphere and modality. J of Neuroscience 18 (4): 1559–70.

9) Mahncke HW, Connor BB, Appelman J, et.al. 2006. Memory enhancement in healthy older adults using a brain plasticity-based training

program. A randomized, controlled study. Proceedings of the National Academy of Sciences. U.S.A., 103 (33): 12523–28.

10) Schwatrz JP and Mijail D. 2002. The mind and brain: neuplasticity and the power of mental force. New York: Regan Books/Harper Collins.

11) Donaghue JP and Mijail D. 2006. Paralyzed man uses thoughts to move cursor. New York Times July 13.

12) Kandel ER. 2003. The molecular biology of memory storage: A dialog between genes and synapses. Nobel Lectures. Physiology and medicine. 1996–2000. Singapore: World Scientific Publishing. 402.

13) Kandel ER 2006. In search of memory: The emergence of a new science of the mind. New York: W.W. Norton and Co. 166.

14) Kandel ER 1998. A new intellectual framework for psychiatry. American J of Psychiatry 155 (4): 457–69.

15) Etkin A, Pettenger HJ, Polan HJ and Kandel ER. 2005. Toward a neurobiology of psychotherapy: Basic science and clinical application. J of Neuropsychiatry and Clinical Neurosciences, 17: 145–58.

16) Stickgold R, Hobsen JA, Rosse R, et.al. Sleep, learning and dreams: off-line memory reprocessing. Science 294 (5544): 1052–57.

17) Frank MG, Issa NP and Stryker MP. 2001. Sleep enchances plasticity in developing visual cortex. Neuron 30 (1): 275–87.

Chapter 12

1) Aaron P. Nelson, Ph.D. Achieving Optimal Memory. McGraw-Hill N.Y. 2005.

2) Douglas J, Mason, Psy.D. and Spencer Xavier Smith. The Memory Doctor. New Harbinger Publications, Inc. Okland, Califo. 2005.

3) Berloquin, Pierre. 365 Exercises for the Mind. New York, N.Y. Barnes And Noble 1998.

4) Garmon, David and Bragdon, Allen D. Building Mental Muscle. New York, N.Y. 1998.

5) Katz, Lawrence B. and Manning Rubin. Keep Your Brain Alive. Workman Publishing Co. 1999.

6) Parlette, Snowden. The Brain Workout Book. New York, N.Y. Evans and Co. 1997.

7) Albrecht, Karl. Brain Power: Learn to Improve Your Thinking Skills. A Fireside book. Simon and Schuster 1992.

8) Amen, Daniel G. Change Your Brain, Change Your Life. Three River Press. New York, N.Y. 1998.

9) Hubert, Bill. Bal-A-Vis-X. Rhythmic balance/auditory/vision exercises For Brain Body Integration. Wichita, Kansas 2001.

10) Hodgkins P, Boken M, Capone NM, et.al. Office visits and prescription fill rates in patients with ADHD. Program and abstracts of the 19th U.S. Psychiatric and Mental Health Congress. November 15–19, 2006. New Orleans, La.

11) Bateman B, Warner JO, Hutchinsen E, et.al. The effect of a double blind placebo controlled artificial food colourings and benzoate preservative challenge on hyperactivity in a general population sample of preschool children. Arch. Dis. Child. 2004: 89: 506–511.

12) Boris M and Mandel FS. Foods and additives are common causes of the Attention deficit hyperactive disorder in children. Ann. Allergies. 1994: 72: 462–468.

13) Carter CM, Uzbanowicz M, Hemsley R, et.al. Effect of a few food diets on attention deficit disorder. Arch. Dis. Child. 1993: 69: 564–568.

14) Jensen PS and Kenny DT. The effects of yoga on the attention and behaviour of boys with attention-deficit hyperactivity disorder (ADHD) J Atten Disord 2004: 7: 205–216.

15) Konafal E, Cortese S, Lecendreux M, et.al. Effectiveness of iron supplementation. 2005: 116: e732–734. Life Style and Complementary Therapies for ADHD. Summary article-Medline.

16) Arnold LE, Bozzolo H, Hollway J, et.al. Serum zinc correlates with parents and teacher-rated inattention in children with attention deficit hyperactivity disorder. J Child Adolesc Psychopharmacol. 2005:15: 628–626.

17) Richardson AJ and Montgomery P. The Oxford-Durhan study: A randomized controlled trial of dietary supplementation with fatty acids in children with developmental coordination disorder. Pediatrics 2005: 115: 1360–1366.

18) Smits MG, VanStel HF, Vander Heijden K, et.al. Melatonin improves health status and sleep in children with idiopathic chronic sleep-onset insomnia: a randomized placebo-controlled trial.

19) Kuo FE and Taylor AF. A potential natural treatment for attention-deficit hyperactivity disorder: evidence from national study. Am J Public Health. 2004: 94: 1580–1586.

20) Sapolsky RM. 1996. Why stress is bad for your brain. Science 273: (5276) 749–50.

21) Hallowell EM and Ratey JJ. Delivered from Distraction. 2006 Ballentine Books, New York. Pgs214–221.

22) Putnam, Stephen C. Nurturing Your ADHD Child with Exercise. 2001. Upper Access Book Publishers. Hinesburg, VT.

Chapter 14

1) Brestan EV and Eyberg MS. 1998. Effective psychosocial treatment of conduct disorder in children and adolescents: 29 years, 82 studies and 5272 kids. J of Clinical Psychology 27 (2) 180–189.

2) Greene RW, Beiderman J, Zerwas S, et.al. Psychiatric comorbidity, family dysfunction and social impairment in referred youth with oppositional defiant disorder. American J of Psychiatry 159: 1214–1224.

3) Biederman J and Wilens TE, Mick E, et.al. 1999. Protective effects of ADHD pharmacotherapy on subsequent substance abuse. Pediatrics 1999: 104 (2): e20.

4) Milberger S, Biederman J, Faraone S, et.al. 1997. Attention deficit Hyperactivity disorder associated with early initiation of cigarette smoking in children and adolescents. J Am Acad Child Adolesc Psychiatry.

5) Barkley RA, et.al. Driving in young adults with attention deficit Hyperactivity disorder: Knowledge, performance, adverse outcomes and the role of executive functioning. J Int Neuropsychol Soc. 2002: 8 (5) 655–672.

6) Barkley RA. Behavioral inhibition, sustained attention and executive Functions: constructing a unifying theory of ADHD. Psychological Bulletin 1997: 121: 65–94.

7) Biederman J, Faraone S, Milberger S et.al. A prospective four-year Follow-up study of attention deficit hyperactivity and related disorders. Arc. Gen. Psychitry 1996: 53: 437–446.

8) Fischer M, Barkley RA, Edelbrock CS, et.al. The adolescent outcome of Hyperactive children diagnosed by research criteria: II Academic attentional and neuropsychological status. J Consult Clin Psychol 1990:58: 580–588.

9) Barkley RA, Anastopoules AD, Guevrement D, et.al. 1997. Adolescent Outcome of boys with attention deficit hyperactivity disorder and social disability: Results from a 4 year longitudinal follow-up study. J of Consult and Clin. Psychology 65 (5) 758–767.

Chapter 15

1) Milberger S, Biederman J, Faraone S, et.al. Is maternal smoking during

pregnancy a risk factor for attention deficit hyperactivity disorder in children? Am Psychiatry 153: 1138–1142. 1996.

2) Cantwell DP. Attention deficit disorder: a review of the past 10 years. J Am Acad Child Psychiatry 35:978–987. 1996.

3) Biederman J. Attention deficit hyperactivity disorder: A life-span perspective. J of Clinical Psychiatry 1998:59 (Supplement 1–13.

4) Klee S, Garfinkel B, Beauchesne H: Attention deficit in adults. Psychiatric Annals 1986: 16: 52–56.

5) Seidman LJ, Valera E, Bush G. Brain function and structure in adults with attention deficit hyperactivity disorder. Psychiatric Clinics of North America 2004: 27: 323–347.

6) Kessler RC, Adler L, Barkley R, et.al. The prevalence and correlates of Adult ADHD in the United States: results form the National Comorbidity Survey Replication. Am J Psychiatry 2006: 163: 716–723.

7) Barkley RA, Fischer M. The ADHD Report Vole 13 Number 6. 2005.

Chapter 16

1) American Academy of Child and Adolescent Psychiatry. Practice Parameters for the assessment and treatment of children, adolescents and adults with attention deficit hyperactivity disorder. J Am Acad Child Adolescent Psychiatry 1997: 36 (10 Suppl): 855–1215.

2) Biederman J, Faraone SV, Spencer T, et.al. Gender differences in a sample of adults with attention deficit hyperactivity disorder. Psychiatry Res. 1994: 53: 13–29.

3) Harvey AS, Epstein J and Curry JF. The neuropsychology of an adult with attention deficit hyperactivity disorder. A meta-analytic review. Neuropsychology 2004.

4) Seidman LJ, Biederman J, Weber, et.al. Neuropsychological function in adults with ADHD. Biological Psychiatry 1998: 44: 260–268.

Chapter 17

1) Beiderman J, Faraone SV, Spencer T, et.al. Patterns of psychiatric-comorbidity, cognition and psychosocial functioning in adults with attention deficit hyperactivity disorder. Am J Psychiatry 1993: 150: 1792–1798.

2) Buchsbaum MS, Haier RJ, Sostek AJ, et.al. Attention dysfunction

and Psychopathology in college men. Arch Gen Psychiatry 1985: 42: 354–360.

3) Heldnack JA, Moberg PJ, Arnold SE, et.al. Speed of processing and verbal learning deficits in adults diagnosed with attention deficit disorder. Neuropsychiatry, Neuropsychology and Behavioral Neurology 1995: 8: 282–292.

4) Biederman J, Faraone SV, Spencer TJ, et.al. Functional impairments in adults with self-reports and diagnosed ADHD: A controlled study of 1001 Adults in the community. J Clin Psychiatry 2006: 67: 524–540.

Chapter 18

1) Spencer T, Biederman J, Wilens T, et.al. 1996. Pharmacotherapy of ADHD across the life cycle. J Am Acad Child Adolesc Psychiatry.

2) Wilens T, Biederman J, Spencer T. Attention deficit/hyperactivity disorder. In Annual Review of Medicine, ed. Caskey CT, 2002: 53: 113–151.

3) Baumgaertel A and Wolraich ML. Practice guidelines for the diagnosis and management of attention deficit hyperactivity disorder. Ambulatory Child Health 1998: 4:51.

4) The MTA Cooperative Group. A 14 month randomized clinical trial of treatment strategies for attention deficit/hyperactivity disorder. Arch Gen Psychiatry 1999: 56:1073–86.

5) Beiderman J, Wilens T, Mick E, et.al. Attention deficit hyperactivity disorder. Pediatrics 104 (2): e20 Aug 1999.

6) Spencer T, Biederman J. (2004) Stimulant treatment of adult attention deficit hyperactivity disorder: Psychiatric Clinics of North America.

7) Faraone SV, Biderman J. Efficacy of Adderall for attention deficit hyperactivity disorder: A meta-analysis. J Atten Disorder 2002:6: 69–75.

8) Kollins SH. Comparing the abuse potential of methylphenidate versus other stimulants: a review of available evidence and relevance to the ADHD patient. J Clin Psychiatry. 2003: 64 (Sppl 11): 14–18.

9) Prince JB. Pharmacotherapy of attention deficit hyperactivity disorder in children and adolescents: update on new stimulant preparation, atamoxitine and novel treatment. Child Adolesc Psychiatry Clin N Am 2006: 15:13–50.

10) Waxmonsky JG. Nonstimulant therapies for attention deficit hyperactivity disorder (ADHD) in children and adults. Essent. Psychopharmacol. 2005: 6: 262–276.

11) Brown RT. Amber RW, Freeman WS, et.al. Treatment of attention

deficit hyperactivity disorder. Overview of the evidence. Pediatrics. 2005: 115: e 749 – e757.

Recommended Reading
1) Delivered from Distraction by Edward M. Hallowell, M.D. and John J. Ratey, M.D. Ballentine Press, New York.
2) The Explosive Child by Ross W. Greene, Ph.D. 2005 HarperCollins publishers, New York
3) The Brain That Changed Itself by Norman Doidge, M.D. 2007 Viking Penguin Group, New York.
4) The Executive Brain by Elkhonon Goldberg. 2001. Oxford University Press. New York, NY.
5) Change Your Brain Change Your Life by Daniel G. Amen, M.D. 1998. Three Rivers Press. New York, NY.

ABOUT THE CONTRIBUTORS

▶ **LYNN GIMPEL, PH.D.**

B.S. in Pharmacy and Chemistry. Graduated Magna cum Laude from Southwestern State College School of Pharmacy, Weatherford, Oklahoma.

Ph.D. in Medical Physiology from University of Oklahoma School of Medicine

Post-doctoral National Institute of Health Fellow at Emory University School of Medicine Department of Physiology

Co-Director: Marriage and Sex Counselling Clinic Emory U. School of Medicine

Director of Medical Education: Advanced Recovery Center Atlanta, Georgia

▶ **AVIGAIL GIMPEL, M.S.**

B.A. in Education. Graduated Touro College, Teachers Degree.

M.S. Touro College Graduate Dept. School of Education, Manhattan, New York

Specialty: Reading and Study Methods, Learning Disabilities

Post Masters Degree. David Yellin Teachers College, Jerusalem, Israel

Feuerstein Int'l Center "Enhancement of Learning Potential" Jerusalem, Israel

Teachers Degree (phase I, II, III) Instrumental Enrichment

Certified to train teachers

Directed Teacher Training Seminar, Jerusalem, Israel

Designed program for cognitive skills and curriculum for language study

Teacher for Etz Chaim High School, Moscow, Russia

Designed "Teaching Methodology" seminar for teachers, Etz Chaim High School, Moscow, Russia

Taught at Beit Yehudit High School, Moscow, Russia

Now conducting Parenting Workshops in the Jerusalem area.

Index